Evolved to Move

of related interest

The Alexander Technique
Twelve Fundamentals of Integrated Movement
Penelope Easten
Foreword by Rosa Luisa Rossi
ISBN 978 1 91208 585 9
eISBN 978 1 91208 586 6

Teaching the Alexander Technique
Active Pathways to Integrative Practice
Cathy Madden
ISBN 978 1 84819 388 8
eISBN 978 0 85701 346 0

Awakening Somatic Intelligence
Understanding, Learning & Practicing the Alexander
Technique, Feldenkrais Method & Hatha Yoga
Graeme Lynn
ISBN 978 1 84819 334 5
eISBN 978 0 85701 290 6

Galvanizing Performance
The Alexander Technique as a Catalyst for Excellence
Edited by Kathleen Juul and Cathy Madden
ISBN 978 1 78592 720 1
eISBN 978 0 85701 272 2

EVOLVED TO MOVE

USING THE ALEXANDER TECHNIQUE TO REDUCE PAIN AND IMPROVE FITNESS

Richard Brennan

Edited by Dr Miriam Wohl

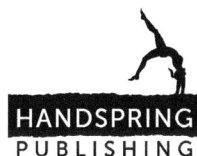

HANDSPRING
PUBLISHING

First published in Great Britain in 2025 by Handspring Publishing,
an imprint of Jessica Kingsley Publishers
Part of John Murray Press

I

Front cover image source: Shutterstock®. The cover image is for
illustrative purposes only, and any person featuring is a model.

A CIP catalogue record for this title is available from the British Library and the Library of Congress

ISBN 978 1 80501 392 1
eISBN 978 1 80501 393 8

Printed and bound by CPI Group (UK) Ltd, Croydon, CR0 4YY

Jessica Kingsley Publishers' policy is to use papers that are natural, renewable and recyclable
products and made from wood grown in sustainable forests. The logging and manufacturing
processes are expected to conform to the environmental regulations of the country of origin.

Handspring Publishing
Carmelite House
50 Victoria Embankment
London EC4Y 0DZ

www.handspringpublishing.com

John Murray Press
Part of Hodder & Stoughton Limited
An Hachette UK Company

The authorised representative in the EEA is Hachette Ireland,
8 Castlecourt Centre, Dublin 15, D15 XTP3, Ireland (email: info@hbgi.ie)

Neck problems are virtually an occupational hazard for Ear, Nose and Throat surgeons. I had serious problems during my working years, but hoped for relief on early retirement. This was not the case and limitation of cervical and thoracic movement became quite an intrusion on my life. Physiotherapy and medication gave only short-term improvement. On being introduced to the Alexander Technique I was somewhat sceptical that anything was going to work, but can only describe the relief gained, and maintained, as quite incredible. General posture has improved, and neck mobility has returned to that last experienced more than twenty years ago. What more could one ask for?

(KIERAN TOBIN, MBBCH, BAO, FRCS(ENG), FRCS(IRL), DLO

PAST-PRESIDENT OF THE IRISH OTOLARYNGOLOGICAL,
HEAD AND NECK SOCIETY

PAST-PRESIDENT OF THE ENT SECTION OF THE
ROYAL SOCIETY OF MEDICINE OF IRELAND)

Contents

Acknowledgements

This book could not have been written without the help of the following people. First to all of my pupils and students who have taught me so much over the years; second to the editorial team at Handspring and Jessica Kingsley Publishers, especially Sarah Hamlin, Sarah Thomson, Laura Savage and Katie Forsythe who were so encouraging from the very beginning. Thank you to my daughter Laoise Brennan for doing the initial editing and suggesting other interesting ways of presenting the material. Thanks also to Dr Miriam Wohl, a medical doctor as well as an Alexander teacher and a respected colleague who sub-edited the text before submission and helped me present the material in a way healthcare professionals could easily relate to. I would also like to express gratitude to my son Tim Brennan for his help with choosing and submitting the images. I would also like to thank Jean M. O. Fischer for help granting copyright permission for quotes by F. M. Alexander and to the following people who helped with the illustrations: Ciaran Brennan, Laoise Brennan and Michaela Wohlgemuth and Paul Cook, editor of *Direction Magazine*. Lastly, I am deeply grateful to all the people who read and gave feedback or actually directly contributed to this book, namely Dr Jack Stern, Dr Glenna Batson, Dr Kieran Tobin, Žiga Repanšek, Kecia Chin, Elisa Asín Senosiáin, Professor Joan Van Dyke, Judith Stern and Ana Milek.

Introduction

Throughout the first half of the twentieth century in the UK, a pioneering and highly effective preventive health-improving technique was gaining momentum. As more and more doctors saw just how effective it was at vastly improving and often helping a wide range of chronic conditions, there were growing calls for it to be part of the standard medical training for all doctors. Most intriguing of all was that it seemed to work best for conditions that conventional medicine had failed to remedy. The name of this work was the Alexander Technique.

Due to the impact of World War II, this endeavour was understandably put on hold for several years, but unfortunately even after the war was over it continued to force the Alexander Technique to very much take a back seat in the medical world for many decades. The sudden abundance of trained physiotherapists following the war combined with the death of its founder, F. M. Alexander, in 1955 seemed to signal the end to this promising renaissance in health.

However, the Alexander Technique did not die out completely. Alexander had trained a small number of pupils who devoted the rest of their lives to make sure this important discovery could live on. In this respect, they did succeed because nearly 70 years later, the Alexander Technique has thousands of Alexander teachers worldwide. Yet, it is only vaguely known to some of the medical profession and is still very much a precious jewel waiting to be discovered.

Today there are thousands of books about movement offering different advice and theories about what will help a painful neck, back or any other physical problem. Unfortunately, this advice is all too often confusing, which can result in frustration on the part of the patient or client. This vast ocean of differing opinions often leaves a person in chronic pain not knowing where to start.

There are, however, very few that attempt to give the reason why back and neck pain is so common in our society today. This book is somewhat different to the other books I have written on the subject as it is written especially for those who work in the movement and fitness industries or in the healthcare services. It has always been my belief that practitioners of conventional or complementary medicine and exercise and fitness instructors need to be working together to help as many people as possible to be pain free, so this book is especially written for those medical and movement professionals to enhance what they already know. When the ideas and principles of the Alexander Technique are added to their own knowledge base and skills, I believe that they will be able to help their patients or clients more quickly, efficiently and effectively. It will also help them to be pain free.

Evolved to Move is based on my own personal journey from being a chronic back pain sufferer for almost a decade to being pain free for more than 30 years, and during that time I have helped thousands of people to be pain free also. It is really important, however, that you do not believe anything that is written down in this book; it is far better for you to explore the ideas and principles so that you can discover for yourself whether or not they work.

During the time I was actively searching for a solution for my back pain, I explored many techniques and methods including physiotherapy, chiropractic, osteopathy, acupuncture, Feldenkrais, Rolfing, Pilates, yoga, tai chi, movement therapy, massage, reflexology, metamorphic technique and Reiki healing. I actually became a massage therapist, a metamorphic practitioner and a reflexologist, but I was still in pain.

Some of the therapies were very useful, while others gave only short-term relief or none at all. Over time the pain got worse and worse and developed into sciatica until eventually I could hardly walk. Most of this book is about what I came to value the most, which was the Alexander Technique. It had an immediate impact as it made total sense to me, because instead of just trying to 'fix' myself it helped me to discover why my problem was there in the first place. When I discovered for myself with the help of an Alexander teacher what was causing the problem, I was then able make a complete and lasting recovery. Since 1989 I have helped thousands of people with a wide variety of physical, mental and emotional issues. In that time, I have often found that what works for one person does not work for another even if they have very similar problems. I often wondered whether, had all those practitioners I consulted known about the Alexander Technique, my time being in pain would have been shorter.

Alexander made his discoveries over 130 years ago and it is important to understand that applying the Technique is a hands-on experience that can never adequately be described in words. You may even be surprised to know that the Alexander Technique is not a therapy or treatment of any kind, and it is possible to combine it effectively with any medical, therapy or movement practice. It is a form of transformative health education, or perhaps re-education is a more accurate description, because it is all about rediscovering how to move with improved thinking, co-ordination, balance and ease – just as we used to do as children. In fact, you can easily apply the Technique to yoga, Pilates and all other forms of exercise or movement. Doing so empowers your patients or clients to help themselves between sessions or treatments. The same applies to any other kind of therapy. It does this by teaching a person how to become aware of, and then eliminate, the habitual thinking and consequent postural habits that underlie many of the aches and pains that people experience in later life. Habits that they have absolutely no idea exist. In fact, they are so unaware of them that they don't even know that there is anything to be aware of!

When I completed my own training in 1989, I looked up the statistics for back pain in the developed countries throughout the world – it was 49% (National Association for Back Pain cited in Enfield Chiropractic Clinic 2000). Recently I looked up the statistics again, 35 years later, and I was amazed to see that this figure remains unchanged (British Chiropractic Association 2018) even though we have more orthopaedic surgeons, physiotherapists, chiropractors and osteopaths and far superior medical equipment than ever before. So very clearly something is not working, and we need to find a different approach to help the millions of people suffering right now. I believe that combining the Alexander Technique with other therapies and exercise programmes is that different approach. Unlike most other methods that advise the person what to do and how to do it, the Technique teaches us what *not to do* and how *to prevent it*.

This book is written in a straightforward and simple way and as such it will also be of interest to anyone who is intrigued or fascinated by the design and function of the human being and wish to know more about themselves.

Life is Movement

Men go abroad to wonder at the heights of mountains, at the huge waves of the sea, at the long courses of the rivers, at the vast compass of the ocean, at the circular motions of the stars, and they pass by themselves without wondering.

(SAINT AUGUSTINE OF HIPPO N.D.)

In physics, motion is defined as 'the change in position of an object over time' (Motion 2024). We are all living on a planet that is constantly turning on its axis while at the same time it is revolving around the sun. All this is happening as our entire solar system orbits around the centre of the Milky Way galaxy. Not only that, but our galaxy itself is rotating at an astounding 2.1 million km/h! So, everything in the universe can be considered to be moving and therefore movement is fundamental to the universe and to all life. But let's come back to Earth for a moment and start to look at how we can look at ways of improving the way we move in all of our daily activities.

During our life we are never still – we blink an average of 15,000 times a day; we breathe around 20,000 times a day; and our heart beats at around an incredible 100,000 times daily. The confirmation that a person is no longer alive is when they are no longer breathing and there is no heartbeat, in other words, when there is no movement. Even though movement is integral to human life, many people are not conscious of their habitual way of moving. Our movements when we walk, run, bend, reach and stand up, and even how we breathe, are primarily habitual. We have all been moving before we had a name or a personality and definitely before we could stand, walk or talk. In fact, every one of us has been moving since before we were born. If a pregnant mother's scan shows no movement of the foetus, the doctors and nurses express great concern for the mother and child. It is often the case that many people start to develop unconscious habits of movement that begin to cause lasting harm.

POSTURE AND MOVEMENT

If you are a doctor or physiotherapist alleviating a patient's suffering, or a physical education teacher, sports coach, yoga teacher or Pilates instructor assisting your student to improve health, fitness and wellbeing, the insights from this book can dramatically improve your own and others' current wellness practices. It can help you to understand why the way your patient or client moves deteriorates as they grow older. This knowledge can assist you in becoming an even better practitioner. Unlike many adults, most young children's movements are upright, free and varied. This book will explore the reasons many of us change this natural way of moving, which I believe is the underlying cause for millions of people suffering with some of the health problems existing today.

The Alexander Technique is a unique method which identifies, considers and then changes habits that are harmful, allowing people to return to good health. It is a process of self-discovery which leads to increased awareness and improved co-ordination and balance. The late Kieran Tobin, an ENT surgeon at the University College Hospital in Galway, Ireland and senior lecturer at the Galway Medical School, publicly advocated in *The Irish Times* (Siggins 2012) far greater awareness of the Alexander Technique for doctors during medical training due to the fact he personally experienced great success with his own neck problem.

Alexander principles highlight common harmful habits which damage and age the body. We adopt such habits unconsciously over time, and they become embedded in all our actions (Figure 1). Through understanding the Alexander principles, you can begin to be aware of the common harmful habits which wear the body out before its time. The Technique is something a person can use on their own to help themselves to move in a way without excessive tension during any activity.

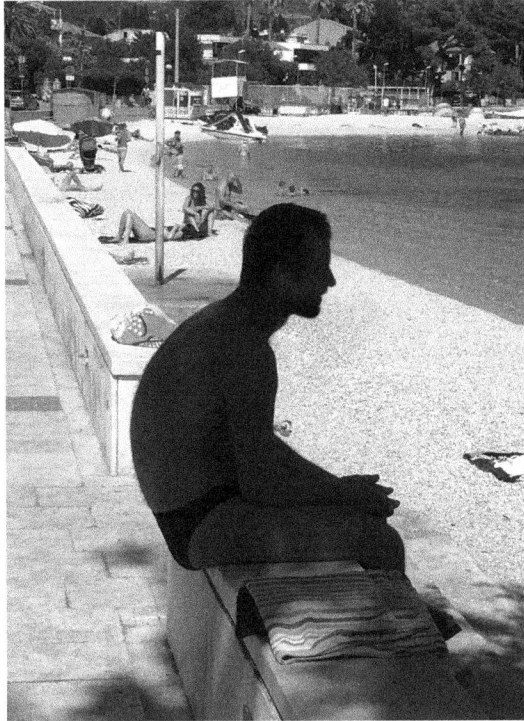

Figure 1: Many people are unaware that the way they sit, stand or move can cause health problems.

What is the Alexander Technique?

Just take a moment to think about how many people come to you with various musculoskeletal problems which occur seemingly without any apparent reason – including backache, neck pain, arthritis, knee or hip problems. As a medical or fitness professional you may often find yourself trying to help your patients or clients without really knowing what has caused the pain or restricted movement in the first place. Nearly half of the population in developed countries have backache alone and have done so as long as I can remember. This is evidence that points to the fact that we still do not understand the fundamental reason why so many millions of people suffer with this condition. Doctors today are diagnosing with very sophisticated equipment to ascertain 'what is wrong' with a person, but rarely do they understand the reason *why* something has gone wrong in the first place (Figure 2). Of course, knowing what is wrong is very helpful, but to my mind knowing why a person's health has gone wrong in the first place can be even more helpful because it expands awareness and self-knowledge in the patient, helping them to let go of the habits at the root of the pain so they can eradicate the pain for good without the use of drugs or surgery.

The Alexander Technique is different from any therapy or exercise programme because it is based on actively learning how to think about performing everyday actions in a different way. The sole purpose of the Technique is to identify any habit which is harmful to a person's general wellbeing. Its methodology is unique because, unlike most systems that advise people *what to do* or *how to do it*, this technique teaches people *what not to do* and *how to prevent harmful habits.*

If we take the comparison of driving a car, it is obvious that the way a person drives is instrumental in the performance of the vehicle. If we use the wrong gear for the appropriate speed, press on the brakes too hard, ride the clutch or drive with the parking brake on, the car will wear out prematurely. It is exactly the same with the human being except for one important factor: the human body automatically repairs itself once the cause of the problem has been removed. Even when in pain, many people rarely consider whether they are 'using' their body well or badly – they just move in a way that feels normal and right to them. Therefore, very few people even realize that they can reduce and eliminate pain by thinking about and then improving the way they move.

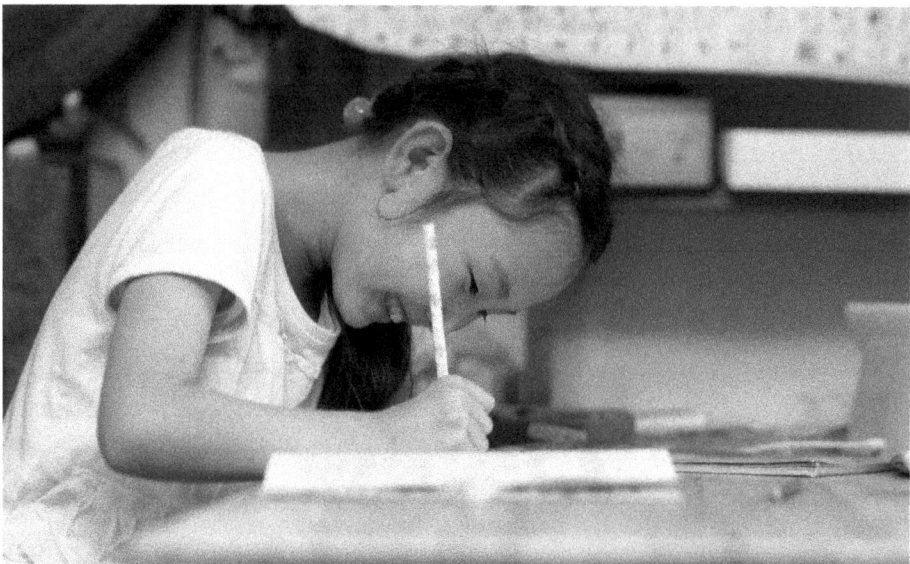

Figure 2: Long hours bending over school desks seriously affect children's posture, which can lead to many of the common aches and pains we see in society today.

A good analogy of this was in an article I read in a newspaper some years ago. An American woman arrived at Heathrow Airport in London from New York. She had arranged to stay with her relatives in Scotland, so she rented a car and proceeded up the M1 motorway. The car was not performing well at all; the engine had no power and could do little more than 30 mph (48 km/h). When the woman got to Edinburgh, she immediately took the car back to the car rental company and strongly complained that there was something very wrong with the car. She reported that it had taken her at least twice as long as expected to get to Scotland and the engine was very noisy and emitted a horrible burning smell. A mechanic checked the car, but could find nothing wrong with it except he admitted there was a burning smell coming from the engine. The woman would not accept the car back and tried to show the mechanic what the problem was. At that point, it became evident that she had never driven a car with gears – she had always driven a car with an automatic gearbox. So, she had driven the car in first gear along the motorway for over 400 miles (644 km) with her foot hard down on the accelerator! She didn't even realize that she needed to change gears! Of course the car was very noisy and didn't go very fast – any car with a manual gearbox would have behaved in exactly the same manner! So, there was absolutely nothing wrong with the car, but there was something wrong with the way she was driving it, which was simply she was not driving the car as it had been designed to be driven.

This amusing story illustrates the fact that when people do not 'drive' themselves in the way they were designed, they start to malfunction. In fact, most people don't even think that they are 'using' anything – they are just going about their daily business. The body is a wonderful 'healing machine' and many unconsciously 'misuse' it for many years before their aches and pains start. In the following chapters we will explore how the human being is designed and how a deeper understanding of the Alexander Technique can enable you to help your patients and clients to become pain free and start to move with the grace and ease that they once had as children, even well into later life.

Transformative education

A very good example of someone who changed the way he moved was George Bernard Shaw. Shaw had been an active man throughout his whole life, but by his mid-seventies he had become slow and was feeling decrepit and, like most other people, just put the changes down to the ageing process. By the time he was 80, however, his balance, co-ordination and general posture were very poor. He had been suffering with a very painful back, stiff neck and shoulders, arthritic hips and knees for years, but now was suffering with angina as well. Each and every step he took was pure agony for him. Several doctors agreed that he was on his last legs and probably had only a few weeks left to live. If he had been living today, he would probably have had artificial hips and knees, but such medical procedures were not available in 1936.

The pain was so bad that he took the advice of a good friend and booked an appointment to see Mr F. M. Alexander who might be able to help even though several doctors could not. When he arrived for his first meeting at 16 Ashley Place, Victoria in London, Shaw could not get up three small steps to ring the doorbell, so he had to ask a passing pedestrian to ring the doorbell for him. At this point he was so frail that he needed three people to help him get up the steps. It turned out that Shaw proved to be the quickest learner of all Alexander's clients. In less than three weeks his pain eased dramatically and he was able to easily walk a mile or more as well as resuming his daily swimming routine. After a course of lessons, he proclaimed himself 'a new man' and everyone around him was amazed to see that Shaw was now moving in a completely different way. In fact, he went on to live another 14 years and died at the age of 94 when he fell off a tall ladder while pruning his trees! Now if you think about it, you don't get many 94-year-olds up ladders in the first place, especially when 14 years before they were unable to get up three steps. In private, he gave Alexander the credit for saving his life and giving him an extra 14 years. Shaw is reported to have said to Alexander, 'I am very grateful to you for restoring me to good health; my knee, hip and back problems are completely cured, and the doctors can no longer detect the angina. I feel like I am moving like a young man again, but you have left me with one problem that I didn't have in the first place; now that I'm 3 inches (8 cm) taller and 2 inches (6 cm) wider in the shoulders, none of my suits fit me any more.' Shaw had to send all his suits back to his tailor for alterations. All through his 80s and early 90s he was known as a 'very sprightly gentleman' and he continued to lead a very full and active life. He publicly declared:

Alexander established not only the beginnings of a far-reaching science of the apparently involuntary movements we call reflexes, but a technique of correction and self-control which forms a substantial addition to our very slender resources in personal education.

(George Bernard Shaw 1950, Preface of London Music in 1888–89)

You may well be wondering how this extraordinary method which caused such a dramatic shift in Shaw's health in a short space of time works; especially at a time before Rolfing had even being developed, and Pilates and yoga were hardly known about. This is exactly what this whole book is about.

Shaw wrote over 60 plays, and he was often over-bending his upper spine while typing, which is exactly what so many people do today at their computers. This habit started to compress his whole body, affecting all the joints in his spine, and the downward pull put enormous pressure on his hips and knees. He also believed that even his angina was caused by poor posture as he was compressing his sternum onto his heart. Alexander first helped Shaw to be aware of his habit and then taught him new ways of thinking about how he sat and moved so that the harmful habits were replaced with healthier ways of being.

The principles that Shaw discovered, based on the discoveries of F. M. Alexander, can be also learned and applied by anyone and are set down in the following chapters. They are very different from therapies or exercise programmes as they are based on actively learning how you perform everyday actions in a different way. The sole purpose of the Technique is to help yourself and other people to avoid doing things in a way that is harmful to their general wellbeing.

CHAPTER ONE SUMMARY
The Alexander Technique is:

- A unique way of understanding how the human being is naturally designed to work.

- A method of heightening our awareness of ourselves and the world around us.
- A way to help patients and clients perform actions in such a way that their psycho-physical equilibrium can be restored.
- A process which helps us to recognize the interferences that people unknowingly inflict upon themselves that affect their natural functions.
- A way to use our intelligence to bring about a desired change so that we may go about our daily activities in a more co-ordinated fashion.
- A way of expanding your level of awareness.
- A technique which a person can practise on their own, to help them to function in a way that causes the appropriate muscle tension at any given time.
- Is a method used to eliminate harmful and unwanted habits.

Evolution of a Technique

Alexander's story of perceptiveness, of intelligence, and of persistence shown by a man without medical training, is one of the true epics of medical research and practice.

(PROFESSOR NIKOLAAS TINBERGEN, NOBEL PRIZE
WINNER FOR MEDICINE AND PHYSIOLOGY 1973)

To fully understand the great number of possibilities that the Alexander Technique makes available, it is essential to understand how Alexander made these discoveries. His problem was not one of pain, stiffness or mobility, but of failure of his own vocal cords! How he overcame his problem himself is truly remarkable by any standards.

VOICE PROBLEM

During the early 1890s, Fredrick Matthias Alexander trained to be an actor in Tasmania, Australia. It was not long before he gained a fine reputation as a first-class reciter, and went on to form his own theatre company specializing in one-man Shakespearean recitals (Figure 3). As he became increasingly successful, Alexander began to perform more often and to larger audiences and was consequently asked to act in larger theatres. With no microphones to help, his voice was under more and more strain, which began to show when he regularly became hoarse in the middle of his performances. He had had respiratory problems from birth, but this problem was different.

He approached a variety of people, including doctors and voice trainers, who gave him medication or various exercises to do, but nothing seemed to make any difference. In fact, the situation deteriorated still further, until on one occasion Alexander could barely finish his recital.

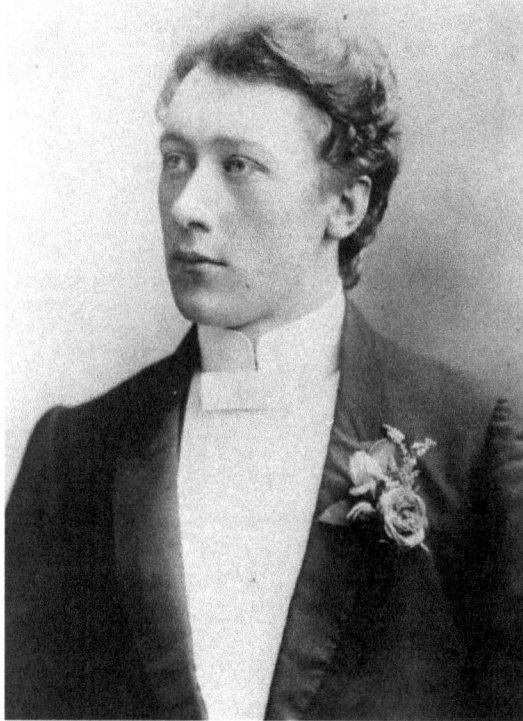

Figure 3: Fredrick Matthias Alexander as a young actor.
Used with permission from Direction Journal

He became more and more anxious as he realized that his entire career was being threatened. Increasingly desperate, he approached his doctor again even though previous treatment had not worked. After a fresh examination of Alexander's throat, the doctor was convinced that the vocal cords had merely been over-strained and prescribed complete rest of his voice for two weeks, advising that this would give Alexander a solution to his problem. Determined to try anything, Alexander used his voice as little as possible for the two-week period preceding his next important engagement. He found that the hoarseness in his voice slowly disappeared.

At the beginning of his next performance, Alexander was delighted to find that his voice was crystal clear; in fact, it was better than it had been for a long time. His delight soon turned into dismay, when half-way through his performance the hoarseness returned just as bad as it was before, and by the end of the evening he could hardly speak. The next day he returned to his doctor to report what had happened. The doctor felt that his recommendation had helped somewhat and advised him to continue with the treatment, but this time for four weeks. What transpired next proved to be at the very core of the Alexander Technique as it is today.

Cause and effect

Alexander refused any further treatment, arguing that after two weeks of following the doctor's instructions implicitly his problem had returned within an hour. He reasoned with the doctor that if his voice was perfect when he started the recital, and yet was in a terrible state by the time he had finished, *it must have been something that he was doing while performing that was causing the problem*. The doctor agreed that this must be the case, but could not explain to Alexander the cause of his vocal problem. Alexander decided there and then that he would just have to find out for himself.

Alexander left the doctor's surgery very determined to find a solution to his curious problem. This took him on a journey of discovery that not only gave him the answer to his question, but also ultimately led him to an understanding of how the body is designed to function and how the body and mind are inseparable. He came to realize that a great many people unknowingly interfere with their own natural movement, contributing to or even causing their own suffering. To take responsibility for one's own health is an essential first step for any patient who wishes to overcome pain or any other health issue. This does not mean they are to blame or 'at fault', the cause is simply something that they are doing that they are unaware of. All too often a doctor, therapist or fitness trainer is unaware, too.

Alexander's logic can be applied to many other conditions that a person suffers from. For example, if someone has no back pain before they do the gardening, yet have back pain after doing the gardening, then it must be that they are unconsciously doing the damage themselves while working in the garden. It is safe to say that this is the underlying cause of many of the problems that your clients or patients have. The same applies to working at a computer, driving or picking up objects. It does not matter what the problem is and what activity might bring it on; there is often an underlying cause, and when that cause is addressed, the problem will gradually disappear.

The first clues

Alexander had only two clues to follow up when he started his investigations:

1. The act of reciting on stage caused the hoarseness and loss of voice.
2. When speaking normally, the hoarseness disappeared, and his voice improved.

Following simple, logical steps, Alexander deduced that if ordinary speaking did not cause him to lose his voice, while reciting did, there must be something different between what he did while speaking normally and what he did when reciting. If he could only find out what that difference was, he might be able to solve the issue by changing the way he was using his voice when reciting. He used mirrors to observe himself both when speaking in his normal voice and again when reciting, to discern the difference between the two. He observed himself carefully, but could see nothing wrong or unnatural while speaking normally, but as soon as he began to recite, he noticed three actions that were different:

1. He tended to pull his head (skull) back and down on to his cervical spine with a certain amount of force.
2. He simultaneously depressed his larynx.
3. He also began to suck air in through his mouth which produced a gasping sound.

Up to that point, Alexander had been completely unaware of these habits. When he observed his speaking voice a second time he noticed similar tendencies, but to a lesser extent, which explained why they previously went undetected. So, Alexander's first discovery was:

> The interference with the body's mechanisms often occurs habitually and unconsciously.

He returned to the mirror with new encouragement and recited again in search of more clues. He noticed these three tendencies became accentuated when reading passages in which unusual demands were made on his voice. This confirmed his earlier supposition that there was a definite connection between the way in which he recited and the strain on his vocal cords.

A maze of questions

Alexander was still unsure of the root cause of his harmful habits and he found himself lost in a maze of questions as to whether it was the sucking in of the air while inhaling that caused him to pull his head back and to depress his larynx, or perhaps it was the depressing of the larynx that caused the sucking in of the air and the pulling back of the head, or perhaps it was the pulling his head back that caused the other two.

After further experimentation, he realized that he could not directly prevent the sudden drawing in of air while inhaling or the depression of the larynx, but he could, to some extent, stop pulling his head back. When he did this, he found that the pressure on the larynx and the sudden intake of breath became less. At this point Alexander wrote in his journal:

> The importance of this discovery cannot be over-estimated, for through it I was led on to the further discovery of the primary control of the working of all the mechanisms of the human organism, and this marked the first important stage of my investigation.
>
> (F. Matthias Alexander 1985, p. 28)

Alexander's second discovery was:

> The existence of a primary control, which organizes balance and co-ordination of the body.

Alexander referred to the relationship between the head, neck and back as this primary control because it influences many of the workings of the body's mechanisms and makes the control of the complex human being relatively simple. Freedom of movement requires the 'primary control' to be allowed to work without any restriction. If the primary control is working well, it helps all movements to be more co-ordinated and economical.

Alexander continued to experiment. When he prevented himself from pulling his head back, the hoarseness in his voice decreased and his voice became clearer. He returned to his doctor who confirmed that there had been considerable improvement in the general condition of his throat and vocal cords. He now had positive proof that the manner in which he was reciting was causing him to lose his voice, and was convinced that changing the way in which he recited would eventually lead to the end of his vocal problems. Alexander's third discovery was:

> The way in which the body is used invariably affects the way
> it functions.

Unreliable sensory feedback mechanism

Convinced that he was at last getting to the heart of the matter, Alexander continued experimenting to see if he could further improve his vocal function. To counteract the tendency to retract his head backwards, he deliberately put his head forward; however, to his surprise he found that this depressed the larynx just as much. To help him unravel this mystery, he added two further mirrors, one on each side of the original one. When he observed himself again, he saw clearly that he was still pulling his head back and down onto his spine as before, despite his best intentions. Alexander clearly saw that he was doing one thing when he was absolutely convinced he was doing the opposite. He had just made his next discovery:

> The existence of faulty sensory appreciation – a phenomenon
> occurring when a person thinks or feels they are doing a particular
> action, when in fact they are doing a different action.

In other words, he could not rely on his sensory feeling alone to tell him accurately what he was doing. At first, he thought that this was his own idiosyncrasy, but later on, when he started to teach his technique to others, he realized that faulty sensory awareness was extremely common. (Please see Chapter Four for more detailed information.) After this realization, Alexander began to see that his findings now implied the possibility of the opening up of an entirely new field of enquiry as to how to correct unreliable sensory awareness and he was obsessed with the desire to explore it.

Soon Alexander noticed that the way he pulled his head back not only depressed his larynx, but also compressed the atlanto-occipital joint, creating tension throughout his body, which affected his posture and balance. He began to see that when reciting he was also lifting his chest, arching his back, thrusting his pelvis forwards, over-tightening his leg muscles and even gripping the floor with his feet. These were actions that he had never noticed before. Alexander's next realization was:

> A person does not function as a collection of separate independent parts, but as a whole unit, with every part affecting every other part.

Alexander remembered that during his acting training he was taught to 'take hold of the floor' with his feet by one of his tutors. He had followed this advice by tensing his feet and toes, believing that his teacher obviously knew better than him. Similarly, your clients may have been told to sit or stand in a certain way in order to correct their posture. Even if they are able to achieve what they thought was being asked of them, they often make the situation worse instead of better. They assume other people know what good posture is, when in fact many do not. Alexander realized that the tightening of all the muscles in his legs and feet were part of the same habit that was causing him to tighten his neck muscles. The habit of 'taking hold of the floor' with his feet had become so ingrained by then that he was completely unaware that he was doing it and he found it almost impossible to recite without all his habits. Alexander saw that:

> A given stimulus produces the same reaction over and over again which, if it goes unchecked, turns into habitual behaviour. This habitual reaction will eventually feel normal and natural to us.

Directions
Based on this last realization, Alexander questioned how to consciously direct himself while reciting. He recognized that he never gave any thought to the way he moved. Instead, he moved in a habitual manner that felt right

to him. Alexander understood that trying to correct bad habits by deliberate action resulted in even more tension, such as pushing his head forwards and up in order to counteract his tendency of pulling his head back and down, which only tightened his neck muscles even more. Alexander tried a different strategy: he experimented with just *thinking* of his head going forwards, and realized that he merely had to think of the directions in order to bring about a change. The meaning of the word *direction*, as Alexander used it, is the process involved in projecting messages (thoughts or instructions) from the brain to the physical mechanisms of the body, so that the muscles would respond to what he told them to do rather than be allowed to work by habit alone. To be clear, a direction or order is something you just think or imagine – it is *not* something you physically do! For example, if one of your patients or clients is hunching their shoulders, you can ask them to 'think' or imagine their shoulders moving away from their ears or from one another. This thought can cause their shoulders to release the tension and therefore become more relaxed. A more detailed explanation of this concept can be found later on in this book (see Chapter Eight).

After Alexander had practised the new directions (thoughts) of allowing his neck to be free so that his head could go forwards and up many times, until he was au fait with those thoughts, he returned to the mirrors to see if this had made a difference during the action of reciting. However, he found that he still failed far more often than he succeeded to stop his head going back and down onto the cervical spine. He believed his own shortcoming prevented him from achieving his objectives, so he searched for possible causes of his failure to stop his head retracting backwards. He realized he was giving his directions successfully right up to the time of reciting, but then reverted back to his old habit of pulling his head back as soon as he opened his mouth to speak. He called this moment 'the critical moment'– this is the moment when it is most likely that a person's automatic habit returns.

He reflected on his goal-oriented approach to reciting and how his attempts to 'get it right' had resulted in tension in his neck muscles. Alexander called this tendency to become fixated with a goal, without considering the process, 'end-gaining'. His next challenge was to find a way to become less fixated on his goal. Alexander allowed a space between the stimulus to speak and the action of reciting. He called this process 'inhibition', a deliberate refusal to react in the usual way, but to use new directions, and by doing so he was able to notice his physical and mental habits more clearly and thereby change the way he used his head and neck and vocal cords.

The above-mentioned principles and techniques he formulated, which primarily consist of awareness, eradication of harmful habits and free choice, form the basis of what we know today as the Alexander Technique. Through diligent practice he freed himself from the harmful habits which had affected his voice and jeopardized his career, and cured himself of the recurring breathing problems that had afflicted him since birth. He returned to his acting career and soon fellow actors who were suffering from similar voice problems approached him for help. He started to teach them what he had learned. Later on, doctors started to refer patients to him, and he soon acquired a very good reputation for helping people when no one else could (Figure 4).

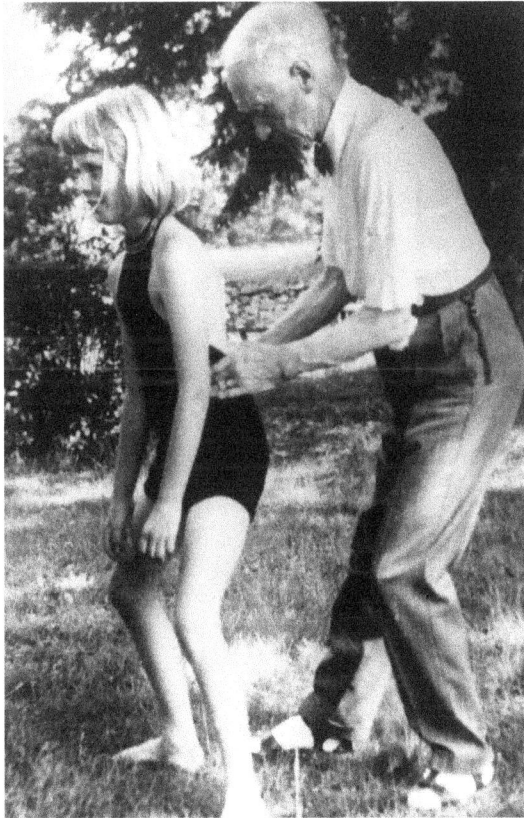

Figure 4: Alexander helping his pupil to restore balanced alignment of the head.
Used with permission from Direction Journal.

CHAPTER TWO SUMMARY

- Interference with the body's mechanisms (poor posture) often occurs habitually and unconsciously.
- Alexander discovered the existence of a primary control, which organizes balance and co-ordinates the movements of human body.
- Alexander also discovered that many people are suffering with an unreliable sensory appreciation while still and during movement.
- The human organism does not function as a collection of separate independent parts, but as a whole unit with every part affecting every other part.
- A given stimulus producing the same reaction over and over again eventually turns into habitual behaviour and starts to feel normal and natural.
- To change a habit that involves muscular tension we need just to *think* of what we what the muscle to do rather than actually changing it by using even more tension.
- Directions – to change a habit that involves muscular tension we need to just *think* of what we what muscles to do rather than allowing them to work habitually.
- Inhibition – to refuse to react habitually to a stimulus.
- Eliminating 'end-gaining'; by inhibiting and directing we can pay attention to how we prepare to perform an action and not be focused on the end result.

CHAPTER THREE

Just Neurons Firing

Change involves carrying out an activity against the habit of life.

(F. MATTHIAS ALEXANDER IN FISCHER 2000, P. 9)

As we saw in the last chapter, Alexander had absolutely no idea he was pulling his head back so forcefully that it was interfering with the functioning of his vocal cords. In my experience of over 35 years, unconscious habits are often the reason behind a multitude of health issues for which people have approached me for help. Exactly like Alexander, they are completely unaware of their detrimental habits. By becoming aware and choosing to change these habits, their daily lives are transformed. As it is far easier to spot someone else's habit than one's own, as a medical or movement professional, with some training you will certainly to be able to help them identify some of these habits and possibly refer them to a fully trained Alexander teacher.

Many of our conscious and unconscious movements are caused by neurons firing in the central nervous system. This process of neurons firing allows the nervous system to communicate by means of electrical impulses and neurotransmitters. These impulses then tell muscle fibres to fire. This in turn contracts the muscles which move the joints and cause the bones to move. As we have 206 bones, 651 muscles and over 300 joints, it would take a huge amount of energy if we had to think about all of these muscles and joints working, especially as we often use different muscles and joints at the same time. If we had to think consciously about every movement, and work out which muscles to use for a particular movement and how much tension to apply, it would take so much time and effort that we would hardly get anything done. Even cooking a simple meal would take hours. This is why habitual movement is very useful – if we repeat an action often enough, neurons start to fire even when we start to think about an intended action, which helps us to move more quickly and efficiently.

Think back to when you learnt to do something new such as driving a car. It was fairly hard and tiring at first, but the more you practised the easier it became. When I first learnt to drive, I consciously had to think of each and every movement when changing gear. First, I had to take my foot off the accelerator and then I put the clutch down. Third, I had to find out what gear I was in and move the gearstick into the desired gear. Last, I had to concentrate when bringing the clutch up to biting point as I pressed down on the acceleration. At first this process took as long or longer than you are taking to read this. By the time I had completed the action, the car had come to a standstill and stalled. Though repetition, all the separate actions involved in changing gear eventually happened habitually and could be performed in only a second or two. The same thing happens to any action when it is repeated often enough; our movements become easy and familiar until we no longer need to think about them.

It is the same as learning to play a musical instrument or any other tasks we learn through repetition. People need to form habits in order to function. However, some habitual movements are healthy, while others are not, and those that are detrimental begin to cause pain or limit movement.

It is important to note that no movement is incorrect or wrong, yet the way we make certain movements can cause pain. Painkillers numb the pain, but they provide only temporary relief, because repetitive habits continue to damage the body whether or not the person feels the pain. Essentially, taking painkillers without remedying the root cause of the pain is like painting over a crack in a wall. Another solution offered to patients is exercise. Unfortunately, the patient will often perform exercises with exactly the same habit which caused the problem in the first place. Last, the patient might resort to manipulation or surgery, but what good is that long term if the person hasn't changed the detrimental habit in the first place? The problem will eventually reoccur. Although medication, exercise, manipulation and surgery can be useful, they can be much more effective if used in conjunction with removing the original cause of the patient's problem.

The rightness and feeling of comfort of a habitual movement can easily be demonstrated if you fold your arms. If you ask anyone if they tend to fold their left arm over their right or vice versa, they probably cannot tell you without actually performing the action even though they have done it countless times before.

You can try it for yourself now:

EXERCISE 1

Fold your arms in whichever way feels usual, normal and comfortable to you. Now look at the two figures below and see which one resembles your habit (see Figures 5 and 6).

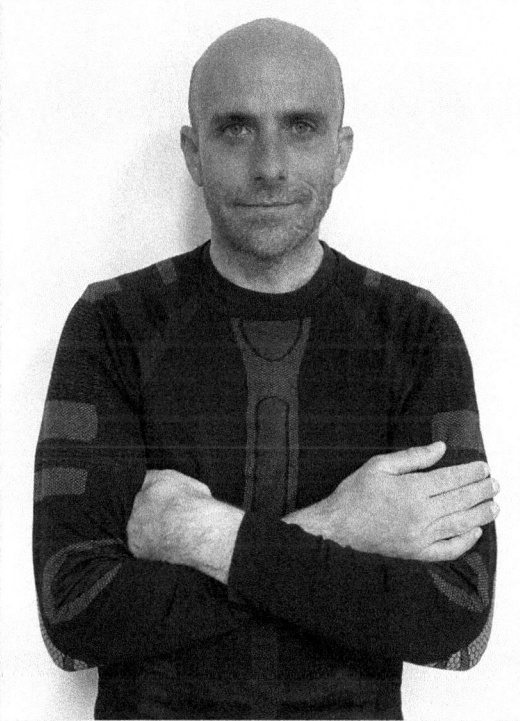

Figure 5: Folding arms in your habitual way feels easy, normal and correct.

Now swap your arms around. If your left forearm was above your right, switch so that now your right forearm is above your left or vice versa. Most people can fold their arms immediately when they perform this action habitually, yet can take up to 15 seconds to fold them non-habitually. Some even find it impossible. Furthermore, the non-habitual way often feels uncomfortable or strange. (It should be noted that a small percentage of the population fold their arms both ways in which case both will feel normal).

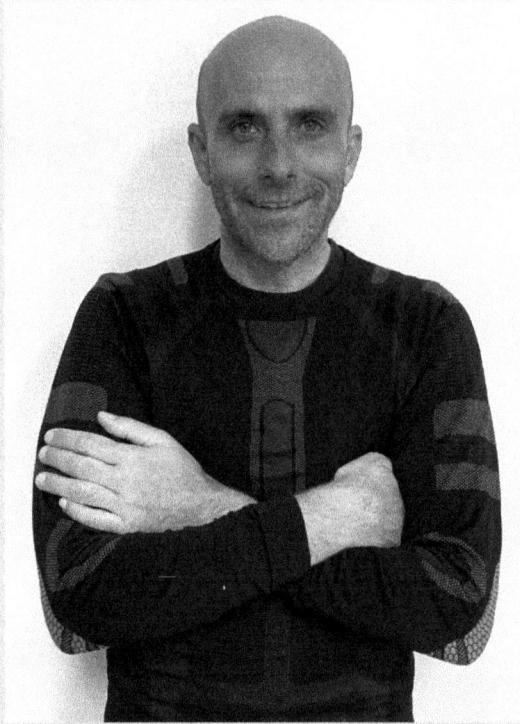

Figure 6: Folding arms in your non-habitual way often takes longer and feels strange.

Folding your arms one way or the other rarely causes pain or discomfort, but many habits do. So, let's look at a common standing habit. Many people tend to lean more on one leg in such a way that they tend to 'sink' into one their hips (see Figures 7 and 8). This is often an unconscious habit, so the one hip they favour will be consistently under more pressure than the other, and consequently the hip joint will wear out sooner. This not only causes damage to the hip joint, but also places the knee and ankle joints under strain and can cause problems there, too. Next time you are queuing in a bank, post office or supermarket, observe those waiting in front of you to see if they are standing evenly or are pulling down into one of their hips.

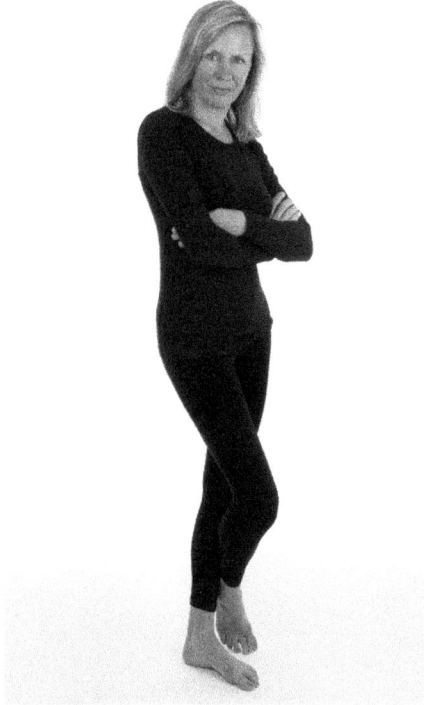

Figure 7: Many people stand in an unbalanced way, causing wear and tear on the hip, knee or ankle joints.

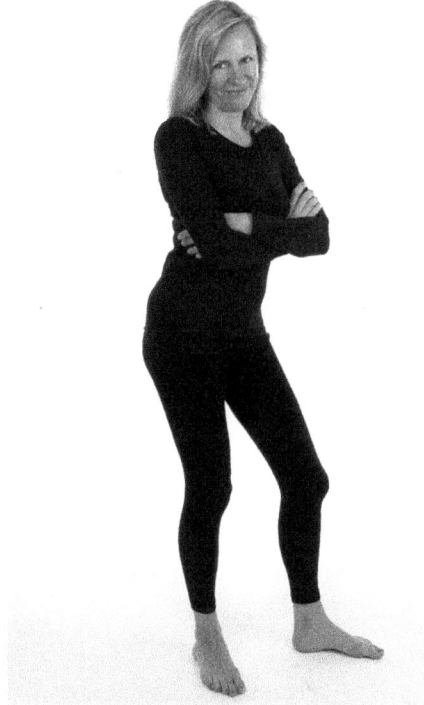

Figure 8: Misaligned ways of standing are very common in developed countries.

You can try this for yourself as well. While standing, lean into your left leg and then into your right. Does one or the other feel more comfortable? If so, you have just discovered a potentially harmful habit. If any of your patients, clients or students suffer from a hip, knee or ankle problem, this is a very helpful awareness exercise. Though the awareness that the Technique makes available, a person can consciously distribute the bodyweight evenly through both feet.

In his first book, *Man's Supreme Inheritance* (2002), Alexander suggested a simple solution to the detrimental habits that people have when standing which can be taught in a few minutes; his advice was to put the feet slightly apart with one foot behind the other (see Figure 9). This can help to bring the rest of the body back into balance and I have found it to be very effective to many people with back pain when standing for long periods.

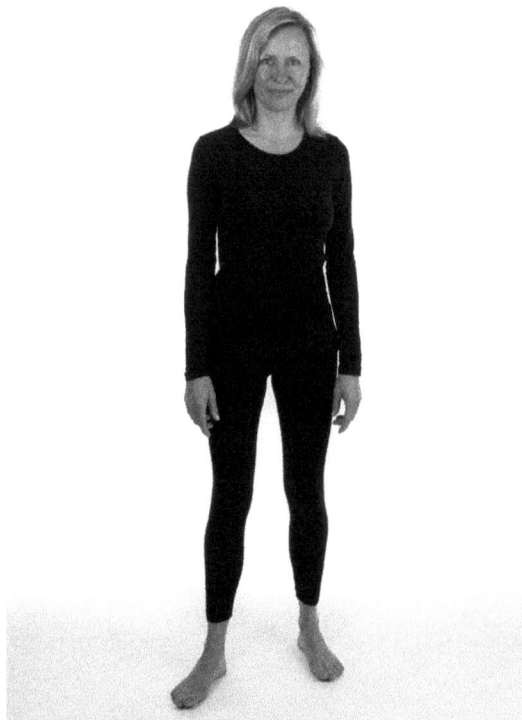

Figure 9: Alexander suggested standing with the feet apart and one foot slightly behind the other to achieve a balanced posture.

MY BACK PROBLEM

I am writing not only from the point of view of someone who has been effectively helping people with health issues for over 35 years, but as someone who suffered with chronic back problem myself. I know, from personal experience, what it is like to be in pain for a long period of time. Indeed, that is what drew me to the Alexander Technique in the first place. My back pain was primarily caused by sitting twisted in a car all day long in my occupation as a driving instructor. I often spent over 60 hours a week sitting in a car and before long I developed lower back pain. At first, it manifested as occasional backache which could be relieved by a massage or some gentle exercise, but before long I was suffering with a condition so painful that at times I could hardly walk.

My father was a medical doctor (GP), so I asked him for advice. Although he was concerned about my condition, he could offer me little help other than painkillers and the standard medical advice at the time, which was rest. This provided temporary relief, yet as time went on even powerful painkillers became less effective. I had a young family at the time, so I needed to return to work due to financial pressures. Sitting in the car for hours was the worst possible position as it exacerbated the pain. Since I was raised in a medical family, I was referred to the best physiotherapists and although a few treatments helped for a day or two, my condition steadily worsened. The exercises and lumbar roll I was given seemed to aggravate the pain. I also began to suffer from sciatica pain shooting down my left leg and before long I could not sit, stand or walk without pain throughout my body. It felt as though I was being stabbed repeatedly with a sharp knife!

Eventually, I was referred to one of the best orthopaedic surgeons in the UK at the time; he took X-rays and performed a number of tests. I was eventually diagnosed with three severely prolapsed discs, but no one told me what had caused the discs to be prolapsed in the first place, or how to realign the vertebrae and relieve the pressure on the discs. I was offered pain management and was told that I would never be able to live a normal life again. I was dissatisfied with this outcome because I did not want to 'manage' my pain – I wanted to be free of it!

The pain was worsening so I consulted another surgeon who advised me to undergo surgery to completely remove the three lowest discs (L3-L4, L4-L5 and L5-S1) because most of them had been worn away and I was told that there wasn't much disc left anyway! He also advised the fusion of lumbar vertebrae 3, 4 and 5 to reduce the level of pain.

As reducing the pain level was exactly what I wanted, I agreed to the operation, but my father persuaded me to cancel the operation, because as a general practitioner he had treated patients who had undergone similar operations, many of whom were in more pain than ever before and very few who were any better. As a last desperate attempt to find some relief from the pain I underwent a one-week intensive course of physiotherapy treatment, even though this had not worked before. I became an in-patient at a large residential physiotherapy hospital near London, UK. One of the treatments at the hospital involved improving posture and I was told to 'hold myself straight' and 'pull my shoulders back', but this only aggravated my pain instantly, in fact it seemed to aggravate the pain of all the other patients in the session, too. Although the physiotherapists were doing their best to help, the treatment and exercises they gave me were not helping me at all. When I was discharged from the hospital, my back pain was worse than ever, but I had exhausted all the avenues orthodox medicine had to offer and was left none the wiser about the reason for the wear and tear to the discs.

At this stage, I started to investigate various forms of complementary medicine. At first, I tried the more established therapies such as chiropractic, osteopathy, homeopathy, massage and acupuncture, and later less orthodox treatments such as reflexology, metamorphic technique, aromatherapy, Reiki and spiritual healing. I was so desperate at that point I that would have tried almost anything. While some treatments reduced the pain to some extent, I could only get short-term relief as the severe pain always returned within days of any treatment. I finally gave up after many years of searching and resigned myself to a life of pain. Up to this point no one, including myself, had any answers as to why the discs had prolapsed in the first place, especially since I was still in my twenties at the time.

By chance, I met an Alexander teacher who explained that the Alexander Technique is effective in alleviating back pain when other remedies had been unsuccessful. I had no idea what it was and was understandably sceptical after all the other treatments had failed to solve my problem. Nonetheless, I decided to have a couple of sessions to see what it was all about. At this point I had nothing to lose, because the pain was present day and night. I had no idea what 'learning and practising the Alexander Technique' entailed. I had heard that the Technique helped musicians and actors, but I could not really see how it was going to benefit me since I was neither.

Within minutes of my first lesson, my Alexander teacher, Danny Reilly, asked me whether I always sat the way I was now sitting. To be honest I didn't understand what he was talking about, and I responded a little defensively: 'What do you mean?' He informed me that I was leaning way off to the left with my left shoulder pulled forwards. I told him frankly that he was mistaken, and I was perfectly straight. Instead of replying he calmly placed a mirror in front of me and I could see clearly that I was twisting to the right while leaning at least 20 degrees to the left exactly as he had said. Despite the fact that I was sitting very crookedly, I felt perfectly straight. This was quite a revelation to me. I was amazed that I had never noticed it before and even more amazed that no one else who had tried to help me had noticed it either. He then made a few gentle adjustments to the way I was sitting, and two things happened: in my new position I felt completely twisted and tilted far to the right but my back pain completely disappeared for the first time in years. He showed me my sitting position in the mirror and to my amazement I saw that I was sitting perfectly straight effortlessly.

After a few lessons, the changes in my posture felt less strange and I began to be pain free for longer periods of time. During one lesson I realized that when I had been teaching people to drive, I needed to see both the road ahead and look to the right to check that the learner drivers I was teaching were looking in their mirrors. So I had developed the habit of leaning to the left while twisting my pelvis to the right. Over the years this had become a habit I 'slipped into' whenever I sat while eating a meal or watching TV. This very habit was at the source of my pain. As the tension continued to subside throughout the series of lessons it was not only my back that improved; I started to sleep better, my self-esteem and confidence grew, and I gradually became happier as well. Within three months, I was leading a normal life again and was lifting, bending and sitting in the car without any pain. Sitting the same way repeatedly had created neural pathways and the neurons in my brain had repeatedly sent the same messages while at the same time another part of my brain had been urging me to stop what I was doing. In other words, my habit had felt 'right and normal' even though I was in tremendous pain.

For seven years I had taken medication, had many massages, practised exercises, yoga and tai chi, had needles put in me, had my spine manipulated over a hundred times, yet all I had needed to do was to change the habit that I had unconsciously adopted. I dread to think what would have happened if I had undergone surgery. I would probably have been in pain for the rest of my life. Instead, I have been pain free and leading an active life for over 35 years. That's the difference the Alexander Technique made to my life. I had seen some of the best doctors (my own father had an excellent reputation), physiotherapists and all kinds of movement experts, and not one of them had commented on my habit of leaning and twisting to the left. This was what prompted me to sign up for the Alexander teacher training programme, because I realized that there must be a lot of people who were in similar situations to me, and I wanted to make a difference to those people.

Learning and applying the Alexander Technique opens up a journey of personal discovery. People can discover exactly what is wrong, and they can learn to reduce pain by simply developing different neuronal pathways by refraining from repeating the habit which is causing the problem. Pain is simply the body's warning system trying to tell us that something is wrong. By being more aware of the principles of the Alexander Technique you can often be more aware of the underlying reason for the problem that people come to you with and, as a result, you will then be in a better position to help them. This does take time so perhaps Mark Twain made a valid point when he said, 'You can't break a bad habit by throwing it out of the window. You've got to walk it slowly down the stairs' (Reader's Digest 1975).

CHAPTER THREE SUMMARY

- We all have habitual ways of moving which are caused by the same neurons firing.
- We are usually unconscious of those habits.
- Our habits are always present in all our activities; however, certain habits may cause pain.
- A detrimental habit is often the root cause of pain and immobility.
- Habits feel 'normal and natural' even though they cause pain and discomfort.
- Often medical and movement professionals do not see these habits simply because they have not been trained to do so.
- With the knowledge obtained in this book, you will be able to spot them and refer patients to help more effectively.

Unknown Unknowns

One of the most remarkable of man's characteristics is his capacity for becoming used to conditions of almost any kind, whether good or bad, both in the self and in the environment, and once he has become used to such conditions, they seem to him both right and natural. This capacity is a boon when it enables him to adapt himself to conditions which are desirable, but it may prove a great danger when the conditions are undesirable. When his sensory appreciation is untrustworthy, it is possible for him to become so familiar with seriously harmful conditions of misuse of himself that these mal-conditions will feel right and comfortable.

(F. MATTHIAS ALEXANDER 1985, P. 82)

The former US Secretary of Defence, Donald Rumsfeld, once said:

There are known knowns; these are things we know we know. We also know there are known unknowns; that is to say we know there are some things we do not know. But there are also unknown unknowns – the ones we don't know we don't know.

('THERE ARE UNKNOWN UNKNOWNS' N.D.)

It is easy to make a list of the things we know – for example, most people know how to talk, walk, sing, read write, make coffee and check their emails along with millions of other things. The list would be far too long to write down in this book! The list of things we know we don't know would be a long one, too. We know that we don't know how to drive a tank, pilot a submarine, or fly a space shuttle or a fighter jet. We know we don't know how to play every musical instrument in the world or how to travel in time. However, if we tried to make a list of all the things that we are not even aware of, there wouldn't be any list at all! Unknown unknowns are things that we are so unaware of that we have no idea of their existence. Much of this knowledge or information would not make much of a difference to your life. However, the unknown unknowns in the area of health and wellbeing can greatly assist you in transforming your life as well as changing the lives of the people who come to you for help.

Unknown unknowns are very common occurrences when driving, often known as blind spots. A blind spot is an area where the driver is completely unaware of its existence until something unexpected happens to expose it. When a blind spot is revealed, the driver would often experience it as a car coming out of nowhere. The learner driver becomes aware of blind spots through repeated exposure. In this chapter we will explore common blind spots in the area of health and wellbeing which are practically universal.

Many of us also have postural blind spots. We may be standing, sitting or moving in habitual ways that we are completely unaware of. These habits can often cause or exacerbate a variety of health problems. A good example of this occurred when a woman came to see me complaining of a sharp pain in her right knee. She had been to the doctor who had sent her for an X-ray and other tests. When she returned to the doctor, he informed her that she had developed arthritis of the right knee. She asked the doctor as to what could have caused this and he answered that as she was 55, it was probably just normal wear and tear. She replied that she was very confused, because she has two knees and as far as she was aware they were exactly the same age. 'How is it,' she asked, 'that one is worn and torn and the other is perfectly healthy?' To my mind, that was a very good question. During her Alexander lessons we discovered that when standing, walking and rising from a chair, she would always favour the right leg, putting undue pressure on the knee joint. When she was able to change this habit, the pain started to ease and after a few weeks it was gone completely.

FAULTY SENSORY APPRECIATION

In Chapter Two we discussed how Alexander's habit of pulling his head back caused him to lose his voice. To counteract this habit, he tried to put his head forwards and up, but this only resulted in him pulling his head back and down to a greater extent. He clearly saw in the mirror that he was actually doing the exact opposite of what he had intended. Like most people, he had relied on his faulty sensory awareness to inform himself about what movements he was making or what position he was in. At first, he thought this habitual blind spot he had stumbled upon was just his own individual defect, but when he started to teach his work to others, he soon realized that the same unreliable sensory experience that he had also affects the majority of people in modern society. He termed this experience *faulty sensory appreciation*. In short, we think we are doing one thing when in fact we may be doing something very different from what we feel we are doing.

SENSORY FEELINGS

I want to be clear that the sensory feelings that Alexander discovered were unreliable did not include any of the five senses of sight, hearing, smell, taste and touch, nor was he talking about emotional feelings. He was referring to the kinaesthetic and proprioceptive senses. The word *kinaesthetic* is an ancient Greek compound of *cineō* (which means motion) and *aesthēsis*, which means sensation. The kinaesthetic sense uses input receptors from within the muscles and joints; it also sends messages to the brain whenever there is movement. These sensations send impulses along nerves to the brain, and thus inform us of movement that the body is making. The word *proprioception* comes from two Latin words: *proprius*, meaning 'one's own', and *percepio*, meaning 'to gain, learn, perceive or understand'. It is the sense that informs us of the relative position of parts of the body in relation to one another at any given moment in time. Like the kinaesthetic sense, it is referred to as an internal, or interoceptive, sense, because it is information from within the body itself. Kinaesthesia is actually proprioception during movement, and both are extremely important for co-ordination, balance and overall posture. It is these inter-oceptive senses that Alexander discovered to be faulty or unreliable. In his book *The Use of the Self*, Alexander wrote:

> This shows how confident I was, in spite of my past experience, that I should be able to put into practice any idea that I thought desirable. When I found myself unable to do so, I thought that this was merely a personal idiosyncrasy, but my teaching experience of the past 35 years and my observation of people with whom I have come into contact in other ways have convinced me that this was not an idiosyncrasy, but that most people would have done the same in similar circumstances. I was indeed suffering from a delusion that is practically universal, the delusion that because we are able to do what we 'will to do' in acts that are habitual and involve familiar sensory experiences, we shall be equally successful in doing what we 'will to do' in acts which are contrary to our habit and therefore involve sensory experiences that are unfamiliar.
>
> *(F. Matthias Alexander 1985, p. 31)*

A NEW POSSIBILITY

Once Alexander realized he was unable to trust his sensory feelings alone as to what movements he was making, he saw an entirely new field of enquiry open up before him. In my own experience with back pain, the concept of faulty appreciation was not taken into account by any health professionals I visited at the time, or at least, I wasn't made aware of it. I never thought for a second that it was possible that I was causing my own back pain by the way I performed my daily activities.

Although someone may feel sure that they have a certain posture or are moving a particular way, these positions or movements can feel very different to the reality. It is not until they see themselves in the reflection of a mirror or shop window or on video that they realize how different their posture is from the way they feel it is.

Alexander's discovery about faulty sensory appreciation puts many methods for improving health, wellbeing and fitness training into question. It suggests that many of the vast number of people involved in sport, doing workouts, practising yoga or martial arts or all the other forms of exercise are possibly doing those activities in a potentially harmful way. Perhaps this is one of the main reasons why so many sports and exercise injuries occur every year.

There is nothing wrong with any form of exercise, but it is the manner in which people perform them that can cause the problems. The yoga or Pilates instructors I have talked to over the years often explained that when they demonstrate a posture or movement, many of their students move differently from how they had been instructed to move. While students can believe they are copying the instructor, their faulty sensory appreciation prevents them from accurately replicating the posture or action.

> The right thing to do would be the last thing we should do, left to ourselves, because it would be the last thing we should think it would be the right thing to do. Everyone wants to be right, but no one stops to consider if their idea of right is right. When people are wrong, the thing that is right is bound to be wrong to them.
>
> (F. MATTHIAS ALEXANDER IN FISCHER 2000, P. 32)

Over the last 35 years I have talked to many doctors, physiotherapists, fitness and sports instructors, yoga and Pilates teachers, manual handling trainers and ergonomic instructors. I have found that very few were aware of faulty sensory appreciation. This is extremely important, because you may be giving your patients or clients a series of beneficial instructions, but they may be performing them incorrectly. In the process, they may be exacerbating the very problem they asked you to help with. The following awareness exercises can give you a practical experience of unreliable sensory feedback.

EXERCISE 2

1. Stand in a room with lots of space around you and close your eyes.
2. Lift your right arm up to horizontal to the side.
3. Now lift your left arm up to horizontal to the front.
4. How did you sense your arm moving?

Your kinaesthetic sense allowed you to feel the movement.

EXERCISE 3

1. Stand in a room with lots of space around you with a long mirror in front of you and close your eyes.
2. Lift your right arm up to the side so that it *feels* horizontal with your palm facing down. Hold it perfectly still.
3. Repeat with your left arm and again hold it very still.
4. Open your eyes and look in the mirror to see whether your arms were both horizontal.

Note: if you don't have a mirror, you can do this with a friend and a camera; ask them to take a photo of you from all angles before you open your eyes. You can also try this exercise with clients.

One of the most common examples of the faulty sensory appreciation is evident when asking a person to stand up straight. When people feel they are sitting or standing up straight they are often leaning backwards from the waist. It is apparent that the boy in Figure 10 is not straight, but in fact he is leaning backwards. If you told him he was not straight he probably would not believe you, because he feels completely straight.

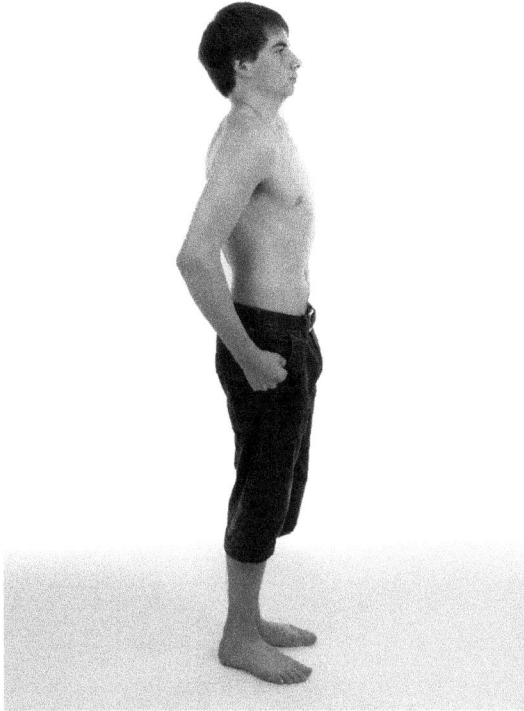

Figure 10: Trying to stand up straight increases the muscular tension and often causes a person to over-arch their back. This can cause or exacerbate lower back pain.

Usually, people don't give any thought as to how much tension their muscles are using as they move; they simply move in the way that feels *normal* and *right* to them. Yet this is the main problem; as I have said already, people's habits invariably feel totally normal, comfortable and right to them, even though they may be experiencing pain. This is due to the nervous system habituation.

Another good example of an instruction that is often interpreted incorrectly that I often come across in my practice is one that people use when bending or lifting. During manual-handling courses a common instruction when lifting a person or heavy object is *bend the knees and keep the back straight.* It is common to misinterpret this instruction to mean *keep the back vertical.* So many nurses and care workers I have met attempt to lift heavy patients while trying to keep their backs vertical, which can result in injury. When young children bend down to pick something up, they bend their knees, hips and ankle joints. Just look at the child in Figure 11: although her back is straight, it is not vertical.

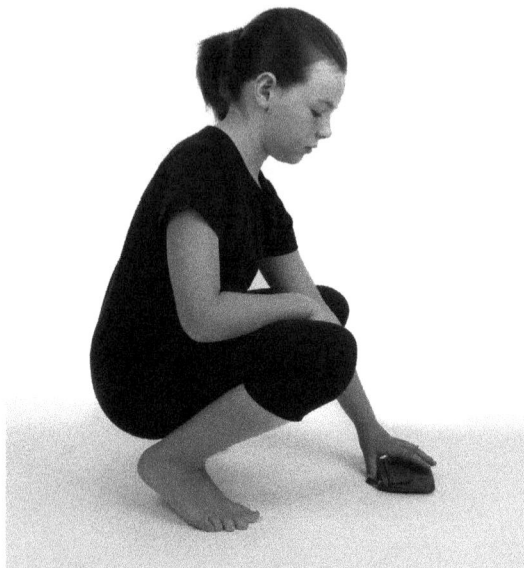

Figure 11: As children we used ourselves in a balanced and co-ordinated way naturally.

There are a few ways to find out what a patient or client is doing to cause pain or discomfort. As a practitioner, you can carefully watch them carry out normal everyday movements to see if you can identify an action that might be exacerbating their pain. By videoing them or sending them for guidance to an Alexander teacher you can obtain reliable feedback in order to make suggestions for a beneficial change. You can try the following two observation exercises at home to gain a practical understanding of faulty sensory appreciation:

EXERCISE 4

1. Stand side-on to a long mirror.
2. *Without looking in the mirror* (using feeling alone), come to an upright position.
3. Stand as straight as you can.
4. Carefully turn your head towards the mirror without moving the rest of your body and check in the mirror to see whether you are straight.

5. If you are not straight, use the mirror to make yourself straight.
6. Observe if you feel straight after correcting yourself and observe the extra tension you had to make during this action.

Note: You can use a second mirror at 45 degrees to avoid moving your body too much when observing.

EXERCISE 5

1. Look straight ahead and *without looking at your feet*, place them approximately 30 cm (12 inches) apart by using feeling alone.
2. Now place your feet parallel to each other using your feeling alone; both feet should be pointing straight ahead.
3. Look at your feet to check whether they are 30 cm (12 inches) apart and parallel.
4. If necessary, look at your feet and place them parallel with one another and 30 cm (12 in) apart.
5. How do they feel when you have made the final adjustment?

BODY MAPPING

Related to faulty sensory appreciation, 'body mapping' is a technique which explores the comparison of a person's mental image of their own body compared with anatomical reality. Our 'body map' is influenced by the way we *think* we are constructed, rather than how we are actually designed. Body mapping was first described by William Conable, an Alexander teacher and professor of cello at the Ohio State University School of Music. He derived the concept of body mapping by observing the way his music students moved while playing their instruments. He noticed that students would often move according to how they *thought* their body was structured rather than according to the anatomical reality. When he was able to show his students how they were actually anatomically constructed, their movement in playing became efficient, expressive, and appropriate for the task required. Barbara Conable then further developed the concept of body mapping by writing books and training others.

While teaching the Alexander Technique to musicians, both William and Barbara realized that there was a great deal of confusion among their music students about how the body worked, particularly regarding the actual position and size of certain bones, joints and muscles. By being educated on how the body anatomically functions, people can learn to change harmful postural habits more quickly. If your patient or client has an incorrect body map, they could be causing themselves harm. Here are a few of the most common examples of this:

Head–spine joint

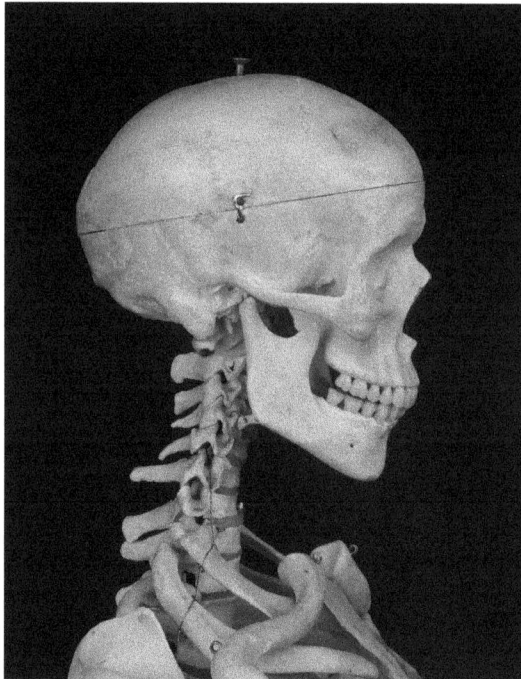

Figure 12: The head is balanced by the spine just below the level of the external auditory canal.

The neck joint is where the atlas and the occiput meet and it is one of the main joints in the body; freedom of this joint is crucial to balance and co-ordination. When asked to locate the position of this joint, many people think it is at the back of the head, or even at the top of their shoulders. In reality the atlanto-occipital joint is located between the earholes (see Figure 12). If a person tries to move the head from the back or lower down if can cause unnecessary muscle tension.

Arm–body joint

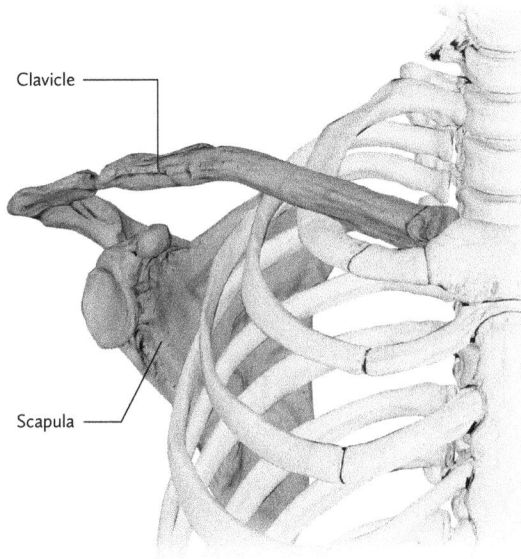

Clavicle

Scapula

Figure 13: The bones of the arm connect to the rest of the body at the sternoclavicular joint.
Source: Kearns, L. (2017) Somatics in Action. London: Handspring. Figure 1.13.

Many people think the arms connect to the rest of their body at the gleno-humeral joint. When we look in the mirror it *appears* that this is where the arms join onto the body. The upper arm (*humerus*) is connected to the shoulder blade (*scapula*), which in turn is connected to the collar bone (*clavicle*). The arm joins the rest of the body where clavicle and the sternum meet. Therefore, the upper end of the arms are very close to each other anatomically. We have five joints in the arm, namely the wrist joint, elbow joint, upper arm to shoulder blade joint, shoulder blade to collar bone joint, and collar bone to the breastbone joint. Yet people often believe they only have three (see Figure 13).

Hip joint

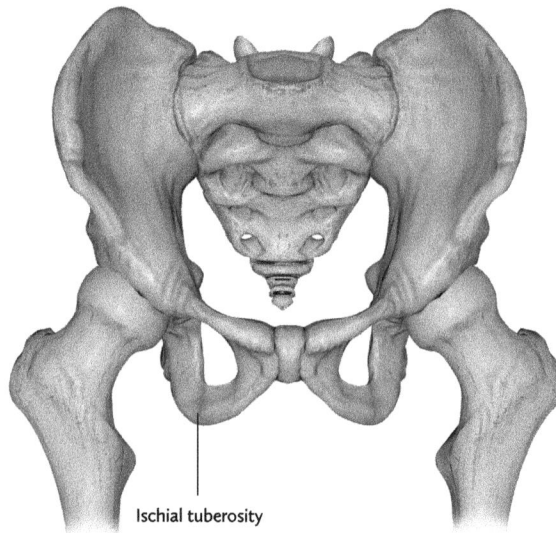

Ischial tuberosity

Figure 14: Many people think the hip joint is located around the iliac crest; however, it is much lower. This can result in people bending their spines instead.
Source: Kearns, L. (2017) Somatics in Action. London: Handspring. Figure 1.16.

It is common for people to think that their hip joint is located at the top of the pelvis, usually in the region of the iliac crest. This is not where the hip joint lies, but it is often where people bend from. As evident from Figure 14, the hip joint is situated lower down and further into the body in the groin area. When some people bend down, however, they will usually try to bend from where they *think* the hip joint is which is very often at the top of the pelvis (the iliac crest). Consequently, they will be bending the spine (around the area of the lumbar fourth and fifth vertebrae) rather than the hip joint. This movement, if repeated enough times, can lead to many lower back problems, particularly around the area of L4 and L5 and the sacroiliac joints, which cause undue pressure.

The spine

If you ask people to draw the shape of the spine many people will draw the spine in a gentle S shape. While this is accurate when standing, the spine actually changes shape depending on what you are doing. When you're sitting or bending the knees, the lumbar area straightens. From the outside it is sometimes possible to observe the back to be completely straight, but the curve still persists on the inside, as can be seen on of an X-ray. When observing a cat, you can see the spine take on different shapes in different situations. When eating its food, the cat's spine is very straight, and when it is lying in front of the fire, its spine is very rounded. When stretching, the cat will arch its back. The human spine also changes shape, depending on what we are doing. Observe how children's spines change while bending or crawling. I have found that the lumbar supports found in cars and back care shops can encourage over-arching of the lumbar spine and can actually exacerbate lower back problems rather than bringing relief.

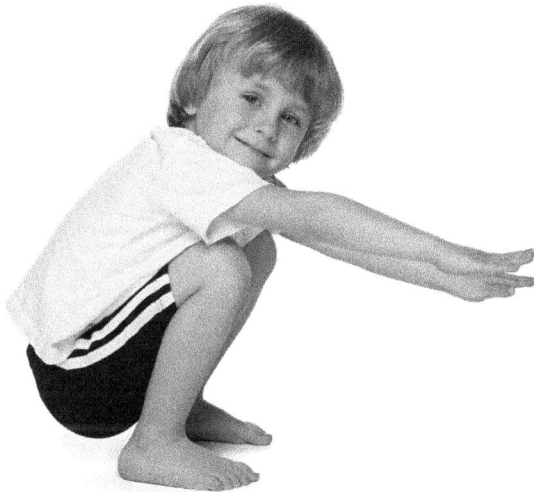

Figure 15: Children naturally keep their spines straight even when bending down to the ground. When the hip, knee and ankle joints are bent the lumbar spine becomes less curved.

The primary action of the spine is for turning or rotary movements rather than bending, which is demonstrated when you observe young children or pre-industrialized people who typically keep the spine long when reaching for something on the ground (see Figure 15). The spine has no hinges, so bending the spine forwards or backwards as though it has hinges can put significant pressure on the intervertebral discs. If this form of spinal movement becomes a habit, it can cause major health problems later in life. The length of the spine is also often miscalculated; it extends from between the earholes to the bottom of the coccyx.

Overall, the key to improving your posture in everyday actions is to become more conscious of what you are actually doing and thinking. Many of us have had incorrect training with regard to posture and movement and that training needs to be corrected. In the next chapter we will have a look at the basic everyday activities.

CHAPTER FOUR SUMMARY

- More knowledge of our faulty sensory awareness in the area of health and wellbeing speeds up the healing process or can avoid injury in the first place.
- People use their unreliable sensory feedback in every movement they make.
- Exercise and movement are often performed with excessive muscular tension, which can cause injury.
- Having a more accurate 'body map' can help people to perform actions more accurately.

Inside Yourself

It has not been realised that the influence of the manner of use is a constant one upon the general functioning of the organism in every reaction and during every moment of life, and that this influence can be a harmful or a beneficial one.

(F. MATTHIAS ALEXANDER 1986, P. XL)

Over the years I have come across misconceptions about the Technique which I would like to clarify. One common example occurs when people hear that I teach the Alexander Technique. Almost without exception they immediately sit bolt upright like a soldier on parade, tensing their muscles in the process. This is because people associate the Technique with good posture and good posture to them means arching their back and pulling their shoulders back as discussed in Chapter Four.

People often think that the Alexander Technique is a cure for back or neck pain and they expect me to carry out certain muscular or skeletal adjustments similar to the way a chiropractor or osteopath works. Yet the Technique is neither a posture-correcting technique nor a remedy for aches and pains. When people learn to stand, sit and move in improved ways, their general posture also improves, alleviating any pains that they might have had. These outcomes are merely consequences of changing detrimental habits and not the fundamental goal of the Technique, which is psycho-physical re-education, and improved posture is a side-effect of the process.

IMPROVING POSTURE

Poor posture not only leaves a person exhausted at the end of the day, but it can also exacerbate or even cause a wide range of muscular problems, poor breathing habits and stiff joints. Misaligned posture can hold you back in almost every aspect of your life. In contrast, good posture can say a lot about a person. People who have a naturally upright alignment appear taller, move more gracefully and subtly emanate confidence, whereas people who hold themselves erect merely look tense and stressed. Posture can be described as the way in which we support and balance our bodies in co-operation with the ever-present force of gravity while we go about our daily activities. It could even be described as an integral part of a person's character The human body is a remarkable 'anti-gravity' mechanism, yet most people unconsciously interfere with its natural mechanisms to such an extent that they obstruct the muscles that are helping to keep us upright. 'Poor posture' is one of the main reasons why many millions of people in industrialized countries suffer from musculoskeletal ailments such as pain, over-tense muscles and stiff joints.

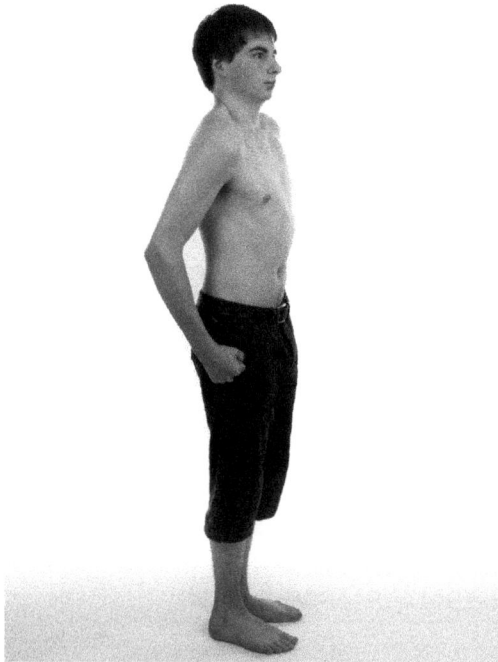

Figure 16: Often people try very hard to maintain good posture.

Few people have been given the tools they need to improve their posture effectively and what I wish to present in this chapter is a fresh approach to improving posture naturally – a way that does not involve physical effort, and a uncomplicated method that everyone can learn. In fact, since we all had wonderful posture when very young it is really something we relearn.

Often the only way people know how to improve their posture is by tensing the entire muscular system (see Figure 16). It is apparent that they are working hard and cannot hold this posture for long. Contrast this stance with the natural-looking, beautiful posture of most young children, who are relaxed while upright, but they are *not doing anything* to be straight. For children, moving in alignment and ease is their natural way of being, they are not 'doing' anything to obtain their graceful posture. It is just *there* because their postural reflexes are being activated without any conscious effort on their part (see Figure 17).

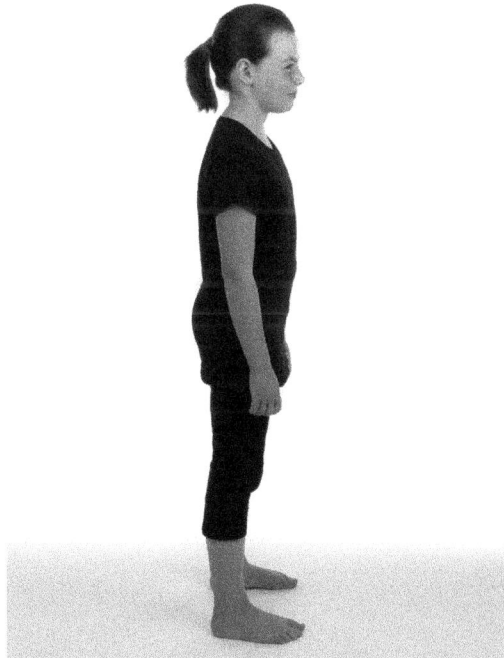

Figure 17: Children naturally have an upright posture without doing anything.

A great deal of postural training for children involves instructions like 'stand up straight', 'pull your shoulders back', 'hold your head high,' 'walk around with a book on your head', 'use this posture aid' or 'do that exercise'. Unfortunately, it is not that simple. Although the order to 'sit or stand up straight' is the most common postural instruction that children are given, it is not an effective command. In my opinion, these instructions only add to the problem, and I believe poor posture or harmful use of themselves is one of the fundamental reasons why a huge number of people are suffering with the multitude of musculoskeletal problems that we see today.

DEFINING POSTURE

When people first try to change their postural habits by using the Alexander Technique, they tend to find it difficult *not* to sit up straight and as a result they tend to over-arch the lumbar curve. In reality it requires far less effort, but it feels strange because is the exact opposite of what many people have been taught to do all their lives. This is another good example of the faulty sensory appreciation that we discussed in the previous chapter. The habit of 'sitting up straight' is often so ingrained that they feel they are doing something wrong when they are not actively 'sitting up straight'. Such detrimental posture training is often given to children at a time when they are easily influenced and do not question the instructions given when they are told to 'straighten up' – they simply obey. I am convinced that this is the reason why many people think improving posture means forcing or tensing the body into different shapes.

Before we start to improve our posture, it is helpful to clarify what we are trying to change. This is perhaps more complex than it first seems, because many people find it much more difficult accurately to explain what the word *posture* means or understand how it can be improved effectively.

In my experience, people tend to define *posture* in one of the following ways:

- The position of my body during various activities.
- The way in which I hold my body.
- The shape that I am in at any given time.
- The way I hold myself.
- The way I carry myself.

- My body's position or stance.
- The position of my limbs and body as a whole.
- The way that I am.
- The way that I hold my body when standing, sitting or moving.
- The way I place my body and limbs.

Just think for a moment – do you agree with any of these descriptions? If not, write down your own definition.

When someone thinks of improving their posture, they generally think of attaining a better shape or position and describing their own posture, usually with the words *hold, position* and *shape*. However, when we think of someone who already has good posture, we often think of young children playing; they invariably move with freedom and grace in a way that has nothing to do with *holding, shape* or *position.*

When people describe their own posture, the phrase that is most often repeated is *the way*. This is because in developed countries most adults have lost the natural movement that they had as children, which is an upright yet free posture and one which involves lots of different shapes and movements. 'The way' simply describes a person's habitual patterns of movement. Just watch young children in a playground as they skip, hop, and walk on their heels or on tiptoes. Their movements are constantly changing, and they do not have a 'set' way of sitting, standing or moving. In contrast, older children and adults 'hold' themselves in unnatural stances and have fixed postural patterns of movement. The habitual patterns of movement of your patients may be easily identifiable to you, but due to their faulty proprioception, they are oblivious of them. Such postural habits that have often been adopted unconsciously can affect mobility and can even lead to physical disability and pain.

REDEFINING POSTURE

Posture is a position or shape as well as the way we move; it is our response to gravity at any given moment. Alexander rarely used the word *posture* as he thought it implied a static position or shape. He preferred the word 'use', which means the way in which we stand, sit *and* move all our bodily mechanisms. He believed that there is no one correct way of moving. Instead, he asserted that there are efficient and harmful ways of moving. Detrimental movements tend to cause health problems if habitually repeated. The natural free posture of young children is the result of a set of innate reflexes known as *postural reflexes*, which are automatic postural responses. These postural reflexes maintain balance and co-ordination, without any conscious involvement. If they begin to lose their balance, their postural reflexes are activated, restoring their co-ordination and poise. The excessive muscular tension many adults have stems from unconscious postural habits which directly interfere with these postural reflexes.

A more accurate definition of the word posture is:

> Posture is the dynamic relationship of one or more parts of the body to the rest.

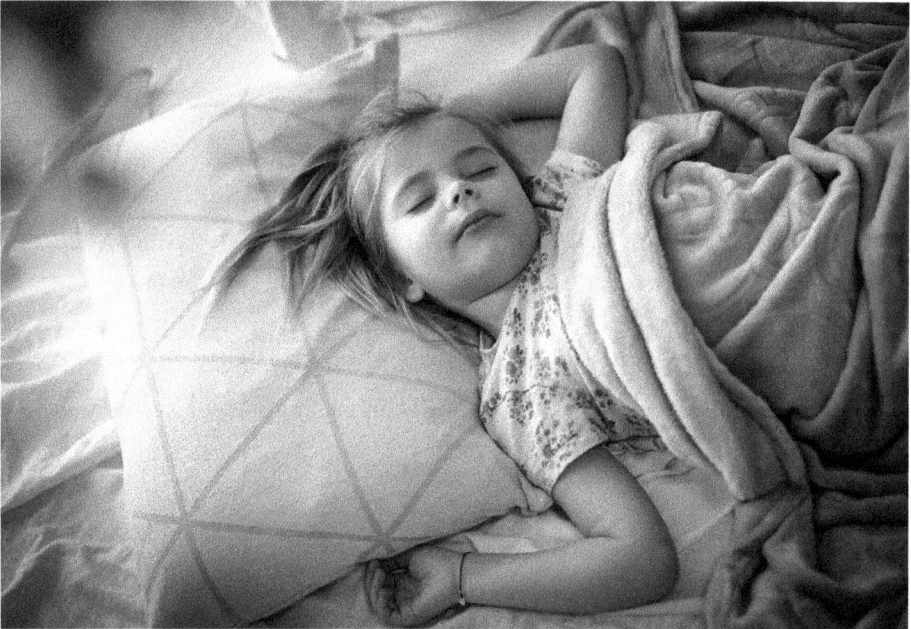

Figure 18: There is no such thing as a correct posture or a correct shape. Good posture requires free movement of all the muscles, bones and joints.

When the relationship is free, good posture happens naturally. When inappropriate muscular tension, collapse or over-extension is present, however, that relationship is compromised and poor posture is inevitable, irrespective of the position or shape. Thus, if we have freedom within the body, the healthy upright posture will be there without us having to do anything. To achieve this, one must first become aware of the excessive and unconscious tension patterns before one can change them. If you look at Figure 18 you will see that while the child's shape is not what most people would call 'good posture', all the muscles are very relaxed so the relationship between one part of her body and another is free.

POSTURAL REFLEXES AND MUSCLES

The most important physical factor when considering posture is how the muscular system functions. This system comprises two distinct types of muscle, each with different functions: postural muscles and phasic muscles.

Postural muscles
These comprise predominately slow twitch muscle fibres whose function is to keep us upright against the ever-present force of gravity. We rarely have to think about maintaining our balance as we go about our daily activities – it is all done for us unconsciously by a system of complex postural reflexes. We can stand for a long time without these muscles tiring because they are 'fatigue resistant' and automatically triggered by a series of reflexes throughout the body. These reflexes send signals to the brain and spinal cord which activate the appropriate muscles. As soon as the stimulus is removed these muscles automatically relax.

Phasic muscles
These comprise predominantly fast twitch muscle fibres which are needed when we perform activities, and work very differently to postural muscles. To raise an arm to a particular height and speed, a conscious decision must be made. These muscles tire more quickly; if a person holds an arm horizontally out to their side, within a short time the muscles will tire and eventually become painful. This becomes clearer when you look at the chart below which compares the different types of muscle and their function.

Summary table: muscle types

Postural muscles	Phasic or activity muscles
These are the muscles that support a person against the force of gravity, primarily designed to maintain balance.	Muscles primarily designed to perform actions. We use these muscles primarily to perform movements.
They have more 'red' (slow twitch) fibres.	They have more 'white' fast twitch fibres.
They are activated by our postural reflexes, which happen without conscious control.	They are usually activated by the conscious mind but can be habitual.
These muscles are fatigue resistant and therefore take a longer time to tire.	These muscles are not fatigue resistant and therefore tire more quickly.

Attempting to improve posture by deliberately sitting up straight and pulling your shoulders back will never work because the phasic muscles that are being activated to obtain the new position will quickly tire. This makes maintenance of what many would consider 'good posture' for any length of time impossible. Even if someone possessed strong will power and was prepared to put up with the discomfort, the muscles would become stiff and immobile, eventually over time causing muscular or skeletal problems.

Instead, the key to good posture is to reduce the tension in the over-worked *activity muscles* so the *postural muscles* can work unhindered as is their normal function. In other words, the muscular system needs to be rebalanced. Alexander once said, 'If you stop the wrong thing, the right thing will happen by itself' (Mouritz 2022). In other words, rediscovering good posture does not involve doing something; it involves finding something that they *have to stop doing.*

Muscles perform two actions, namely contraction (shortening and tightening) or extension (lengthening and releasing). Muscles generally work in pairs: one muscle will contract while the other opposite lengthens to produce movement. If a person's shoulders are rounded, then it can be the muscles in the front of their body (e.g. the pectoralis major) that are over-contracted; this has the effect that the shoulders are pulled forwards and down. Although the issue lies with the over-contraction of the front muscles and thus requires lengthening, people tend to rectify this habit by deliberately pulling the shoulders back, which merely contracts the back muscles (e.g. the rhomboids). Therefore, when people attempt to straighten by 'sitting or standing up straight', they cause the front and back muscles to work against each other like a 'tug of war', which can dramatically restrict the movement of the shoulder. This illustrates how the usual attempt to 'improve posture' can result in an increase of muscular tension, consequently exacerbating the initial problem (see Figure 9).

> The minute you use force to maintain a certain posture, you betray that all is not well with your world. You show the world that your structure and your posture are at war.
>
> (IDA ROLF 1989)

If a person can learn to release their over-tightened muscles, the shoulder will return to its natural state of freedom. So, the first thing a person needs to do to achieve a healthier, more natural posture is to realize that they never ever have to 'sit up straight' again! Instead, they need to become aware and release the tension in the phasic muscles so that the postural muscles and reflexes can start working efficiently again. This release is obtained by using the principles discussed in the following chapters. Furthermore, it is important to identify the factors which caused posture to *deteriorate in the first place*, and to address the root cause. Let us start with one of the major reasons why many people have poor posture in the first place: the classroom.

THE DECLINE OF UPRIGHT POSTURE

Once children go to school around the age of four or five, their movements usually become more restricted as they are required to sit in a chair at their desk for most of the day. Most children sit for more than 15,000 hours during their time at school, which does not include out-of-school activities such as homework, computer games or watching TV. In 2013 the Institute of Medicine in Washington, DC, USA published a report which found that active children 'show greater attention, have faster cognitive processing speed and perform better on standardized academic tests than children who are less active' (De La Cruz 2017). This was backed up by another separate study published by Lund University, Sweden in 2017 (De La Cruz 2017). This study showed that students who had daily physical education, especially boys, performed better at school. Jesper Fritz, a doctoral student at Lund University and physician at the Skåne University Hospital, was the lead author. He claimed that daily physical activity is an opportunity for the average school to become a high-performing school. It is now well known that activity boosts cognitive functioning. For example, exercise stimulates blood-flow to brain cells. There is now evidence that active kids perform better on standardized tests and pay more attention in school. Since movement helps children to learn, it defies common sense to make children sit still for prolonged periods at school. It is not only sitting that causes a problem; it is the type of chair most children have to sit on in school. The reason many children do not like sitting down for long periods is because often they find the chair uncomfortable. I have observed that many school chairs are not suited to the design of the human body. Among other reasons, this is because the seat of the chair is often *sloping backwards* (see Figure 19). A great number of school chairs have been designed in this way and this distorts children's natural upright posture.

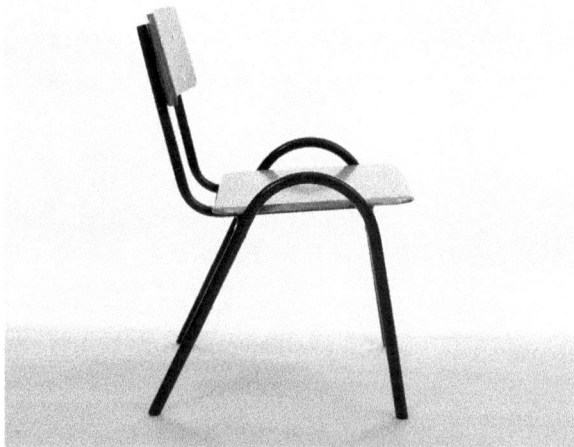

Figure 19: The seat of many school chairs slopes backwards, causing a backward rotation of the pelvis.

Sitting bones (ischial tuberosities) are rounded, so backward-sloping chairs cause the pelvis to rock backwards. This puts them off balance and as a result children need to tense many of their muscles in order to maintain balance. This tension often becomes an unconscious habit that they can carry for the rest of their life. It is my firm belief that this tension causes or exacerbates many musculoskeletal and respiratory problems that we see today. The children feel uncomfortable sitting on the backward slope and within a short time they will try to get up and move around the classroom. In most cases they are immediately ushered back to their chairs. Children have a natural ingenuity and intelligence when it comes to posture and body awareness, and so their next instinctive strategy is to try to counteract the backward slope of the seat by tilting the chair forwards, which raises the back legs of the chair off the floor (see Figure 20). This is an intelligent strategy as it changes the backward slope of the chair seat, making it level or slightly forward-sloping, and helps them to maintain an aligned, upright posture with much less effort. Instead of being inquisitive as to why they do this, most adults just tell them exactly what we were told themselves: 'Don't swing on the chairs – you will break them!' The damage to the child's posture by the backward-sloping chair is usually not considered for a moment.

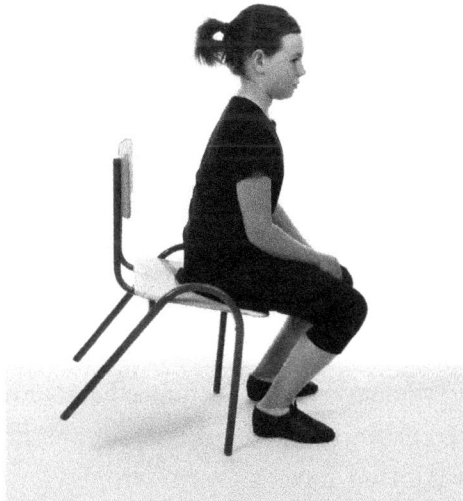

Figure 20: Children develop ways of coping with the backward slope of the chair by tipping the chair forwards.

Children often keep trying to correct their balance and they often develop other techniques to counter the effects of the backward slope, such as sitting on a foot, which raises and supports the pelvis (see Figure 21). This is another method which enables them to pivot on the sitting bones, maintaining an aligned and healthy spine, but this is often actively discouraged in case the blood-flow to the leg is restricted.

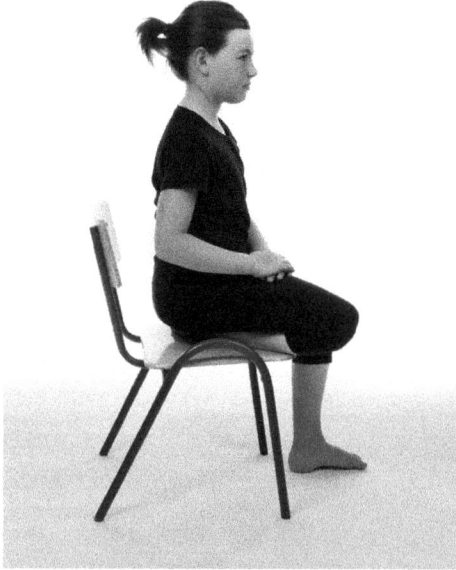

Figure 21: Another strategy for coping with backward-sloping seats is to sit on a foot.

Once they have been prevented from doing what comes naturally to them, children give up, and they learn to endure sitting on backward-sloping chairs for thousands and thousands of hours. Sooner or later, most of them begin to slump as their back muscles become fatigued. To make matters worse, children also have to bend forwards over their desks in order to read, type and write. Since the sitting bones are already rolling backwards, causing the pelvis itself to rotate backwards, the only option left open to them to do this is to bend their upper spines to reach their work. This causes another habit to form which can cause unnecessary wear and tear on the vertebrae and discs, sowing the seeds of future spinal and back problems (see Figure 22).

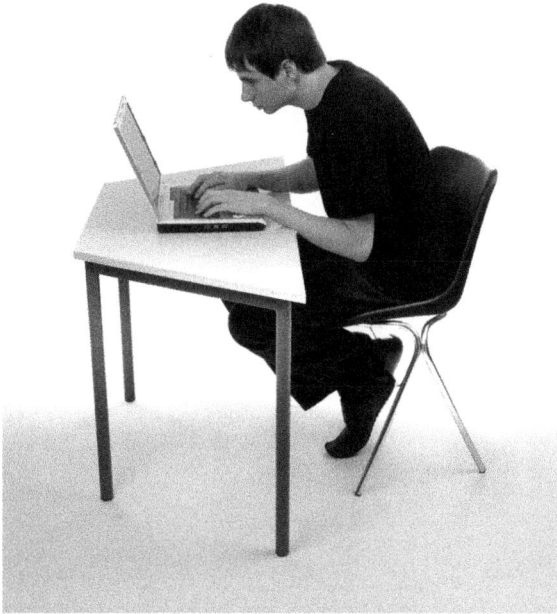

Figure 22: The consequence of the pelvis rolling backwards is that the child has little option but to bend their spine, which becomes a lifelong habit in many of their actions.

The habit of bending forwards from the upper back and neck instead of using the hip, knee and ankle joints becomes lifelong for many people. You can usually see this for yourself if you ask your patient to pick up a pen from a chair or low table; you are likely to see very little movement in the knee or ankle joints. In 2005, the National Back Pain Association reported, 'Research findings suggest that there are several causes of lower back pain in children and adolescents. The most significant seems to be inappropriate furniture at school or in the home. And there's no doubt that inappropriate furniture causes poor posture' (BackCare 2005; see also Mandal 1974; Akerblom 1948; Keegan 1953; Schoberth 1962). In our ignorance, we ruin children's posture by making them sit on badly designed furniture and then we chastize the children for having poor posture. This is not an isolated problem. Just look at any classroom and you will see most of the teenagers working at their desk have rounded backs (see Figure 23).

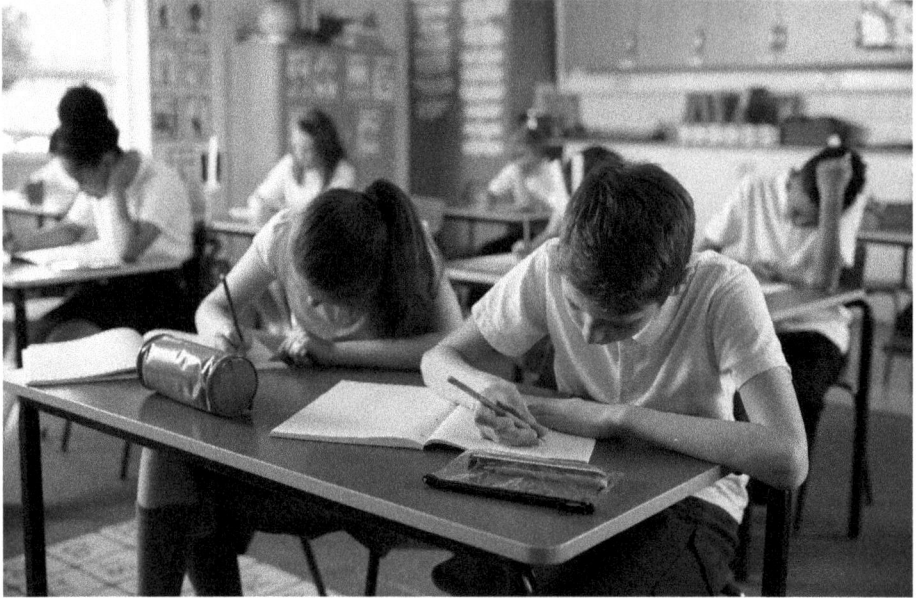

Figure 23: The habit of pulling the head down and bending the spine is practically universal in all schools and colleges.

The chairs used by adults are generally flatter, but not always, so it is likely that your patient may be sitting on backward-sloping chairs for most of the day. If the chair is contributing to the pain, no matter what medication or treatment you prescribe for their back pain it is likely to reoccur. Therefore, one of the first things to do when someone approaches you with a back, neck or hip problem is to check if the chairs they use are sloping backwards. If possible, go and visit their workstation, or ask them to take a photo of the chair. Backward-sloping chairs may be the root cause of their problem. If so, any help you give them will be short-lived because the cause is still present. The problem of backward-sloping chairs and car seats can be rectified by using a simple wedge-shapes cushion (see Figure 24).

It is important to realize that if poor sitting habits have been formed, it is not just a matter of changing a position or a chair; a person also needs to first become conscious of their individual habits and then release the undue tension as well. If from the start of school, a child uses a wedge cushion and writing slope, their natural upright posture can be maintained. It is easy to see the difference between the posture of a child who is using them and one who is not in Figures 25 and 26.

Even if the working chair is flat, the adult often takes the postural habits that they learned at school and college into their working life and would greatly benefit from a series of Alexander lessons.

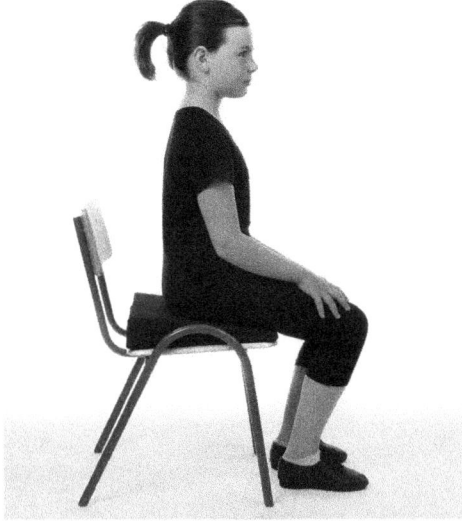

Figure 24: A simple wedge-shaped cushion can help a child to sit at their desk with poise.

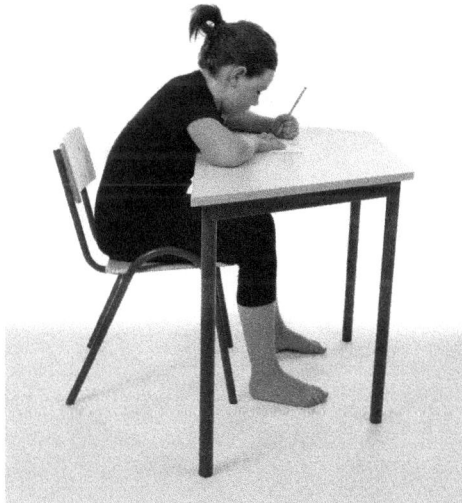

Figure 25: The way a child writes at a school desk is with the head down and the spine bent forwards.

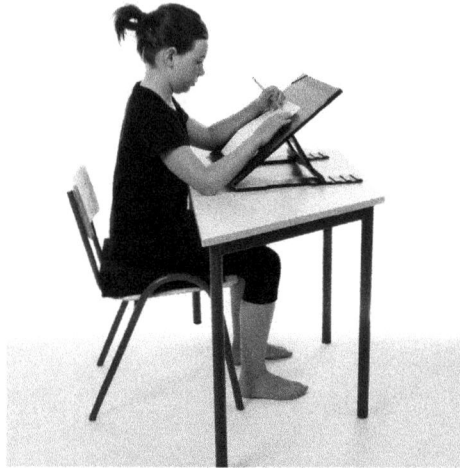

Figure 26: This is the same child working on the same chair at the same desk using a wedge-shaped cushion and a writing slope. Note the difference in the shape of the spine and position of the head.

CHAPTER FIVE SUMMARY

- Alexander preferred not to use the word *posture*, but preferred the word *use* (as in the way we use ourselves) instead, because it included movement as well as position.
- Poor posture often starts in childhood and a major cause is inappropriate school furniture.
- Good posture is innate – but we need to rediscover it.
- Many people try to do something to improve posture, but anything they 'do' will only take them further away from what is natural.
- For a person (with the exception of those with hypermobility spectrum disorder) to obtain good posture or good use of themselves they need to release undue muscular tension in their muscles. This allows the postural reflexes to work more effectively.
- Using a wedge cushion and a writing slope at school can help to prevent poor postural habits from forming in the first place.

The Heart of the Matter

The Alexander Technique gives us all the things we have been looking for in a system of physical education; relief from strain due to maladjustment and consequent improvement in physical and mental health; and along with this a heightening of consciousness on all levels. We cannot ask more from any system; nor, if we seriously desire to alter human beings in a desirable direction, can we ask any less.

(ALDOUS HUXLEY 1938, P. 223)

In this chapter I hope to explain clearly how the Alexander Technique works, but please remember that the Alexander work imparts an experience which is impossible to describe adequately in words, so to really know what the Technique offers it is essential to experience it during a lesson. The Technique can be described as health education or a transformative learning method. In essence it is simple, logical and makes a great deal of sense. Many people's lifestyle today is much more sedentary than that of our ancestors, and this lack of movement can contribute to much of the health problems we see today. When something goes wrong with the body, a person looks to a medical practitioner or health instructor to cure or heal them; they expect the healthcare professions to 'do' something in order to help in the form of surgery, medication, manipulation, massage or supervised exercises. The patient often finds it difficult to grasp the concept that healing can take place when they stop doing or *prevent* something instead of *doing* something. In the same way, when a new pupil comes to me with a health problem, they are expecting me to do something to cure or fix them;

yet this is not how the Alexander Technique works. The body is self-healing, and the Technique simply facilitates this by making the pupil aware that, in many cases, they themselves are hindering the healing process.

> When an investigation comes to be made, it will be found that every single thing we are doing in the work is being done in Nature where the conditions are right, the difference being that we are learning to do it consciously.
>
> (F. MATTHIAS ALEXANDER IN FISCHER 2000, P. 88)

The people who learn the Technique are not called patients or clients, but pupils or students because they are learning how to think and function with improved co-ordination and alignment. Consequently, as the person is able to eliminate the harmful habit, pain or discomfort disappears. Once they realize the cause of their pain, which is usually a particular unconscious habit, they can prevent the habit themselves by changing the way they go about their daily activities. What they learn in an Alexander lesson can also prevent future health problems from occurring in the future. In fact, people do not have to be in pain to benefit from the Technique, they may just want to maintain good health and vitality.

The Alexander Technique is a 'hands-on' technique as the teacher gently touches the pupil, but it is also referred to as non-invasive approach because there is absolutely no force whatsoever during any manipulation or adjustment. The Alexander teacher touches the pupil for four reasons:

1. To find out what habits a person has, because sometimes they are difficult to see and much easier to feel.
2. To bring calmness to the nervous system and consequently to the overly tight muscles.
3. To give subtle messages or 'directions' to help the pupil move in an improved way. Once a teacher discovers the habit that is causing the problem, they will tell the pupil how to initiate the change by inhibiting the habit.

4. To feel when the pupil has released the undue muscular tension.

It is similar to any practical subject that we learn – a diving instructor teaches the learner driver which pedals to press or when to change gears or look in the mirror, then the learner driver repeats the process so often that they can drive the car alone. As with driving, the Alexander pupil is learning to anticipate better, not only on the roads of the town or city, but on the roads of life itself. The Alexander teacher is showing a pupil how *not to do* something! Sometimes the habit may seem very small, but the prevention can make a huge difference. For example, many people tend to pull their heads back and down onto their neck when arising from a chair. Although it is a small movement, it is often done with a great deal of force. When they learn how to release this tension in the neck muscles, their head may only move less than a centimetre (half an inch), but this prevents a powerful downward force onto their spine. Through this small change, the spine naturally lengthens and straightens, which drastically reduces the amount of effort in getting up and thus helps them to move more fluidly and easily. After some lessons they become aware of this habit themselves and are able to activate this lengthening without any help.

> When you stop doing the wrong thing, the right thing does itself.
>
> (F. MATTHIAS ALEXANDER, SEE ADAMS MUSICAL INSTRUMENTS 2014)

DIRECT METHOD

The Alexander Technique operates very differently from most other healthcare methods. By learning the Technique, the person takes responsibility for their own health and vitality. The most fundamental principle of the Technique is to think before reacting to any stimulus. For example, if a person sees in a mirror that their head is leaning to the right, they will probably immediately straighten it, by tightening the muscles on the left of the neck, without much thought. This would be the 'direct way' of straightening the head, however, in all probability, before long that person's head would start to be drawn back to the right again, because the cause of the habit was not addressed. In most cases, a person's head is only pulled to the side due to the contraction (shortening) of the neck muscles on the right side. By immediately correcting the position of the head, the person merely contracts the muscles on the left side, adding even more tension to the neck muscles, which only exacerbates the problem. This is a simple example of what happens when someone is only concerned with correcting the problem, which Alexander called 'end-gaining'.

INDIRECT METHOD

By learning the Alexander Technique, a person would see in the mirror that their head was pulling to the right and first of all prevent the automatic reaction of tightening the muscles on the left side (inhibition) and then they would then work out that the right muscles were pulling the head off balance and would start to release these muscles by just thinking of the right muscles getting longer (directing them to lengthen). When the muscles release, the head naturally becomes balanced again.

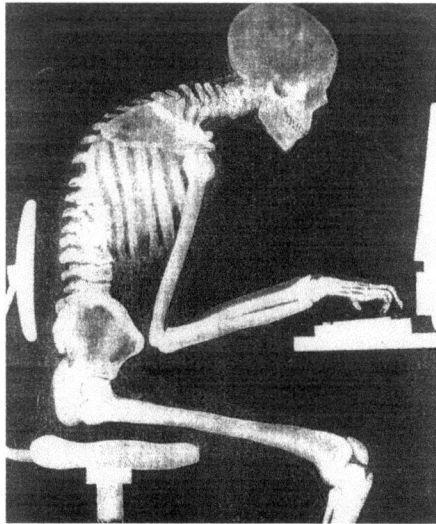

Figure 27: Many people take the habit of bending their upper spine into their adult working life without realizing.
Source: Courtesy of BackCare.

We will look at inhibiting and directing more closely in the next two chapters, but let's look at two more examples of common habits that can lead to harm. The first example is the common tendency to pull the front of the torso down (see Figure 27). This habit can often develop when working at a school desk and it gets stronger if a person does office work. If the person realizes that they have adopted this posture they often 'sit up straight' by contracting the back muscles (see Figure 28). However, these muscles are not the source of the problem. The tension is in the front muscles, such as the abdominal and pectoral muscles (see Figure 29). By just 'sitting up straight' the tension that is the cause of the problem remains unaltered, and then the back muscles are fighting the front muscles resulting in even more tension!

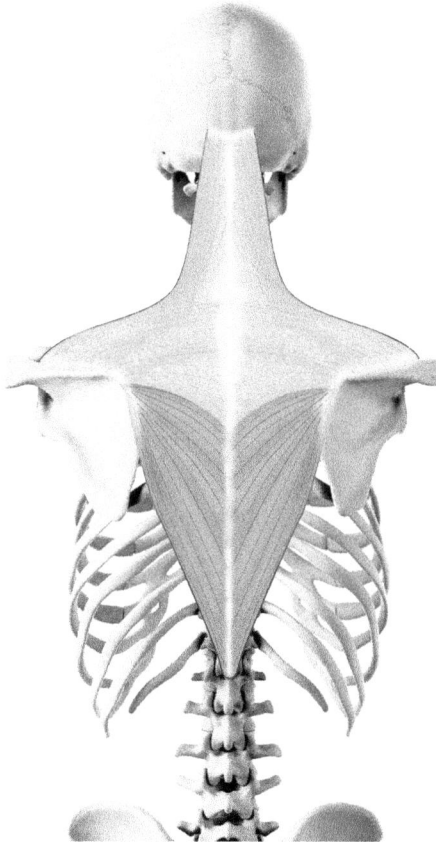

Figure 28: There are 40 muscles in the back alone.
Source: Abrahamson, E. and Langston, J. (2019) Muscle Testing. London: Handspring Publishing. p. 50.

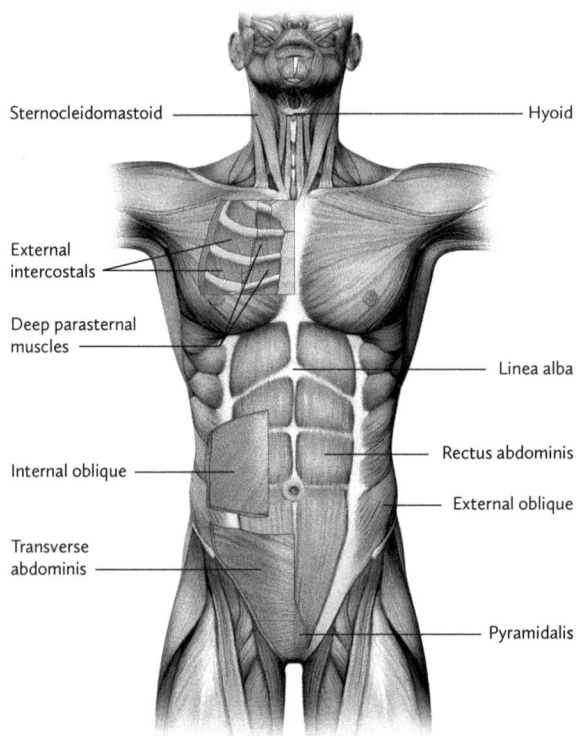

Figure 29: It is often the shortened muscles in the
front that pull us down in the front.

*Source: Black, M. (2022) Centred: Organizing the Body through Kinesiology, Movement
Theory and Pilates Techniques, 2nd edn. London: Handspring. Figure 5.6.*

Practically every person who has ever come to me with lower back pain has
been pulling in their lower back by over-arching the lumbar curve for a long
time due to the fact that they are trying to correct a downward pull in the
front muscles. Once a person is able to release the tension in both the back
and front muscles, the back pain reduces or disappears altogether. People
are usually not aware that they have one set of muscles fighting the opposite
set, they are only aware of physical stiffness, rigidity or pain.

The process of change is a mental process with physical effects; at the
end of the process a person will often not only be pain free, but will be much
more self-aware. This awareness is accompanied by a feeling of freedom and
lightness as the body starts to work as it was designed. On one occasion I
asked one of my pupils, 'What would you like to cover on your lesson today?'
She replied, 'I don't mind; I just want the champagne feeling!' When I asked
her why she called it that; she told me it was because after each session

she always felt so light and bubbly! In essence, a feeling of psycho-physical lightness can be there in all movements when people learn how to allow themselves to move freely. If you were aware of these habits both in yourself and your patients or clients, you would be in a better position to be able to help them. This process does take time, and it is not a quick fix to people's problems, but in my experience, it is very effective as a long-term solution to many health issues.

CHAPTER SIX SUMMARY

The Alexander Technique can be described as health education or a transformative learning method. It works in the following ways:

- Although it is a hands-on technique, the teacher's touch is light and gentle.
- It is completely non-invasive.
- The pupil is healed or cured from a variety of ailments by the natural healing process.
- It works by removing what is causing the health disorder.
- As a person stops moving in a harmful way, the beneficial way of moving happens by itself.
- Awareness is the fundamental principle underlying the Technique.

CHAPTER SEVEN

First Stop and Think

Everyone wants to be right, but no one stops to consider if their idea of right is right.

(F. MATTHIAS ALEXANDER IN FISCHER 2000, P. 69)

This chapter will explore the concept of inhibiting unwanted reactions. Inhibiting is one of the two fundamental skills in the process of changing detrimental habits. As discussed in Chapter Two, Alexander realized that, in order to solve his voice problem, he had to stop his immediate reaction to the stimulus of having to recite. In effect, he was trying so hard to improve his reputation as an actor that he pulled his head back and down onto his neck (and consequently his larynx), causing a loss of voice; he referred to this behaviour as 'end-gaining', which is commonly referred today as being too goal-oriented.

Today this goal-oriented behaviour has become so widespread that, according to a study by the Mental Health Foundation UK in 2018, 74% of people said that the stress they had experienced had made them feel overwhelmed and unable to cope. Stress manifests in daily life in myriad forms such as exam pressure, the daily rush hour, work deadlines and financial and family pressures.

Stress is very infectious. Just as happy or lively people can spread joy with a smile or kind word, many people are also affected by stressful atmospheres. Indeed, we can pick up other people's tension without realizing it, causing us to become irritated with family, friends or colleagues. In fact, stress at work for some is reaching crisis point, as many employees are given large assignments to complete in unrealistic deadlines. This can make people feel that if they are not rushing around feeling panicked or overwhelmed then they are not doing enough. In some cases, if a person refuses to accept extra hours, bosses and colleagues judge them adversely. They are also aware that if they do not 'toe the line' their chances of promotion will be severely affected, or they may lose their job. This mental and emotional pressure is then directly converted into muscular tension, which can be the cause of headaches, back pain, joint problems, overuse injury (commonly called repetitive strain injury (RSI)) or one of the many other common musculo-skeletal problems. The solution is to think, take our time and understand that life is not a series of emergencies.

Without inhibiting, many of your patients will have little or no chance to free themselves of their health problems. At first it isn't easy to inhibit a reaction that has become so familiar, but with practice, it does become easier. When people first give themselves more time, they may well feel uncomfortable at first, because the experience of having time is so unfamiliar. As they cease habitually to rush around, however, they will begin to be more relaxed and have less muscular tension. As a result, they will naturally feel calmer and more able to cope with life.

THE MEANING OF INHIBITION

Over the last 100 years, the word *inhibition* has come to mean the suppression of feelings or the inability to be spontaneous; this was mainly due to the famous psychiatrist Sigmund Freud who used the term in that context. The dictionary definition of inhibition is: 'The restraint of direct expression of an instinct' (Inhibition 2024). If this restraint stems from fear and is unconscious, then it could be seen as being an unhealthy form of suppression and would therefore have a negative connotation. Alexander used the term to mean *deliberately refraining from one's automatic habitual reaction in order to make a conscious decision*. In his book *The Ascent of Man*, Dr Jacob Bronowski (1977, p. 437) claimed, 'We are nature's unique experiment to make the rational intelligence prove sounder than the reflex. Success or failure of this experiment depends on the basic human ability to impose a delay between the stimulus and the response.' This was exactly the subject Alexander was writing about 50 years earlier.

To illustrate the meaning of inhibiting in the work of Alexander, think of a domestic cat chasing a bird or mouse. The cat pauses and waits for exactly the right moment before springing forwards to maximize its chance of success. You could also think of a growth inhibitor: a product that prevents the growth of a plant. So, by inhibiting we are preventing an unwanted automatic habitual and harmful reaction by responding in a mindful and considerate way. It does not mean that people shouldn't move quickly when they want to, but they are not habitually rushing or hurrying. By advising your patients to have Alexander lessons and learning consciously to choose a different way of responding, you can start to help them to bring their lives back towards a more balanced way of living, by learning to take their time as they go about their daily activities, and developing the habit of pausing for a moment so that they consider a way to perform any task with the least amount of tension.

CONSTRUCTIVE REST PRACTICE

This constructive rest practice can help your patients to practise directing and as a result they can become calmer, more aware of the excessive muscular tension they have. It is also known as 'active rest' or the 'semi-supine position'. Regular practice can reduce stress, increase vitality and reduce or eliminate many different aches and pains. Constructive rest also helps to realign the spine and improve overall posture. The best time to practise is either in the morning before work or straight after you finish work. If your clients are at work or out during the day, they can do it when they get back home.

CONSTRUCTIVE REST EXERCISE

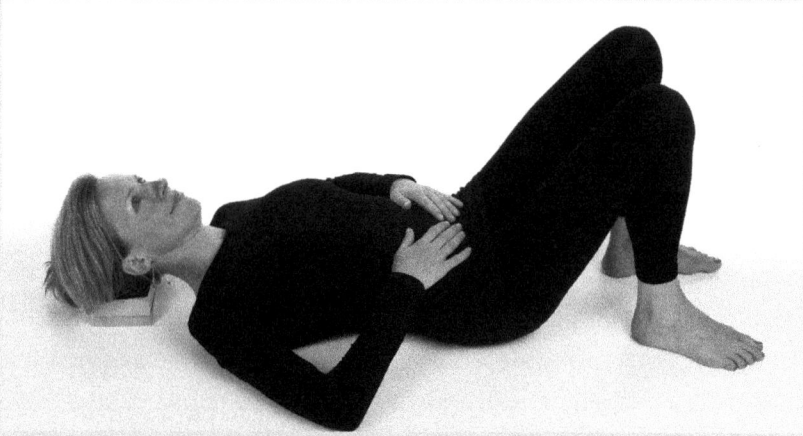

Figure 30: Practising the active rest position every day for 20 minutes can help to release excessive muscle tension and calm the mind.

1. Lie down on your back with some paperback books or magazines underneath your head, your knees bent and feet flat on the floor (see Figure 30).

2. The number of books or magazines beneath your head will vary from person to person, but the head should not be pushed forwards or tilting backwards. If the books or magazines feel too hard, you can place a towel or thin layer of foam on top of the books. Make sure that your head is not falling to the side, retracting backwards or being pushed too far forwards because it is crucial that your breathing and swallowing are unrestricted. The books or magazines are underneath the head to support and to counteract the common habit of pulling the head back, which puts pressure on the neck. Nonetheless, it is still possible to pull the head back when simply lying there.

3. Place your hands each side of the pelvis with the palms facing down or resting gently on either side of your navel.

4. Your feet should be close to your pelvis, but not so near that they are uncomfortable or there is strain in the legs. Make sure that the soles of your feet have even contact with the ground

and that the knees are pointing towards the ceiling. If you find that your legs are falling inwards, or outwards, the following instructions will help to reduce muscle tension in the thighs:

    a. If your legs are falling inwards, then move your feet *closer together*.

    b. If your legs are falling outwards, then move your feet *further apart*.

5. Your back should be resting on the ground, but make sure you do not do anything in order to flatten it. The knees are pointing to the ceiling to enable the lower back (lumbar area) to release towards the floor in comfort; however, this may not happen on the first session. This position helps to straighten the spine by helping to adjust any over-exaggerated curves. This also allows the spinal (intervertebral) discs to absorb fluid and increase their height, which is very helpful for most back problems.

6. Make sure you are lying on a carpeted floor and are warm enough, as it is much harder to release tension if you are feeling cold or lying in a draught. You can place a blanket or duvet over yourself if necessary.

How many books/magazines under the head?

Make sure your head is not tilted back or forwards; if your forehead is slightly closer in the ceiling than your chin you are probably in a good position. If possible, ask an Alexander teacher for advice. You need to be fully alert with your eyes open, which will help you to stay focused and prevent drifting off into sleep. If you do fall asleep, it is a good indication that you probably need more sleep generally. If you find that your mind wanders off, just bring your attention back to yourself and your surroundings.

Benefits

There are many benefits from the constructive rest practice, which include an overall improvement of breathing by helping to release the respiratory muscles and improvement in the circulation system, because blood flows better when the muscles are relaxed. It also reduces pressure on the nerves that may have been trapped due to over-tense muscles. It helps to prevent wear and tear of the bones and joints of the spine and can even rejuvenate parts of the skeleton that have been worn down from misuse of the body. It also allows the internal organs to have more room to function and helps to revitalize and re-energize the body. Last, it brings about an overall reduction in stress and tension physically, mentally and emotionally.

The second part of the process is to learn how to release harmful tension by using mental instruction, which Alexander called 'directing', and these are the topic of the next chapter.

CHAPTER SEVEN SUMMARY

- Stress is one of the main reasons for muscular tension.
- *Inhibiting* is a term that Alexander used to mean mindful thinking before acting.
- Inhibiting helps to increase awareness of any detrimental habits.
- Constructive or active rest can help to calm the muscular and nervous systems.
- Benefits of constructive rest are that it:
  - Allows the intervertebral discs to absorb fluid.
  - Helps to straighten the spine by helping to naturally adjust if the curves have become over-exaggerated.
  - Releases muscular tension.
  - Improves breathing by helping to release the intercostal muscles, the diaphragm and other muscles of respiration.
  - Improves circulation because the blood flows better when muscles are relaxed. Most people find their hands and feet become warmer.
  - Can reduce the pressure on any trapped nerves.
  - Helps to prevent deterioration of the bones and joints of the spine and can even rejuvenate parts of the skeleton that have been worn down from misuse of the body.

- Allows the internal organs to have more room to function.
- Helps to revitalize and re-energize the person.
- Brings about an overall reduction in stress and tension physically, mentally and emotionally.

Thinking in Activity

You come to learn to inhibit and to direct your activity. You learn, first, to inhibit the habitual reaction to certain classes of stimuli, and second, to direct yourself consciously in such a way as to affect certain muscular pulls, which processes bring a new reaction to these stimuli. Boiled down, it all comes to inhibiting a particular reaction to a given stimulus. But no one will see it that way. They will all see it as getting in and out of the chair the right way. It is nothing of the kind. It is that a pupil decides what he will or will not consent to do.

(F. MATTHIAS ALEXANDER IN FISCHER 2000, P. 72)

The other part of the Technique is directing one's activities, which means thinking about the way we do any movement or action. As we saw in Chapter Two, anything Alexander *did* to cure his voice exacerbated the problem, until he tried giving himself mental instructions which he called 'directions'. Directions are purely mental thoughts or instructions which are directly opposite to a person's habit. In his book *The Use of the Self*, he described 'giving directions' as 'A process which involves projecting messages from the brain to the body's mechanisms and conducting the energy necessary for the use of these mechanisms' (Alexander 1985, p. 35).

For example, if someone tends to hunch their shoulders, a direction to counteract this would be 'allow the shoulders to fall away from their head' and not just pull the shoulders back or down. Directions are given before undergoing a particular movement and repeated during the movement itself. Inhibiting gives us the space to allow this to happen. When Alexander gave himself a certain direction, it prevented repeating his habitual pattern of pulling his head back. By inhibiting his usual reaction and then directing, he was able to cure himself of his voice problem as well as a breathing difficulty that had afflicted him since birth.

DIFFERENT DIRECTIONS

Now we are going to look at how to start projecting different directions to bring about a release of tension. It is possible to direct *specific* parts of yourself; for example, you can think of the muscles in your fingers or toes lengthening or the shoulders widening. You can also direct your whole self by thinking of your head moving away from your feet. Alexander often asked his pupils to come to their full height or full stature, and I have personally witnessed most people become taller after releasing tension. It is essential to understand that these 'directions' are only thoughts, because people often try and *do* the directions rather than just thinking them, but this only increases muscle tension.

THE POWER OF THE MIND

The mind is much more powerful than many people realize. This is illustrated by the following account: A woman who lived in Taunton, UK was diagnosed with cancer during some routine tests. Understandably, she became very distraught and anxious, and before long her health deteriorated rapidly, and she was bedridden. As time went on, she became weaker and weaker and visibly suffered all the painful symptoms of cancer. Over several months she felt unable to eat very much and she lost a lot of weight. She was eventually moved into a hospice and her body was dying. At this point, the hospital in Taunton discovered that they had mixed up the records with another patient of the same name – she did not have cancer at all and, in fact, there was nothing wrong with her! When she was informed of the mistake, she immediately started to gain weight and her health quickly returned. This is a clear case of how powerful our mind can be.

The primary direction

Alexander discovered that one of the fundamental causes of poor posture, pain and unco-ordinated movement is an over-tightening of the neck muscles. In the long term, this tends to shorten the spine, causing a downward force throughout the whole body. This affects a person's alignment, balance and co-ordination, causing an over-tightening of the entire muscular system, initiating a vicious cycle. Alexander realized that the priority was to reduce tension in the neck area enabling the primary control to work without interference. *Primary control* is a term used by Alexander to describe the effect on the whole organism of freeing the atlanto-occipital (AO) joint, co-ordinating and balancing the body with the least amount of tension. This allows the body to work as effectively and efficiently as possible. A more detailed account of the primary control can be found in the next chapter. The primary direction which removes the interference of the primary control is:

> Allow the neck to be free *in such a way* that the head can go
> forwards and upward, *in order* that the back can lengthen
> and widen.

Allow the neck to be free

The main purpose of the first part of this instruction is to eliminate the excess tension that is almost always present in the muscles of the neck, mouth and eyes. If your patients or clients want to have effortless and efficient movement the head must have free movement. It is called the 'primary direction' because it needs to be the first direction given; unless the primary control can work without hindrance, all other directions will be relatively ineffective. In the direction 'allow your neck to be free' Alexander referred to freeing the AO joint, which is where the head meets the spine between the earholes as described in Chapter Four. There are several ways to think of this freedom, including allowing the neck to come to 'a quiet or calm place'.

Allow the head to go forward and up

This tells you which way the neck needs to be freed. If you just thought of your neck being free without the thought of an upward direction, the head would probably fall forwards and down towards the chest. It is also important to realize that the movement forwards is often so small that it is hardly detectible. The purpose is to prevent the skull from pulling back and downwards onto the AO joint. This direction helps to keep the head finely balanced, ready to take the rest of the body into movement, allowing the mechanisms of the body to function naturally and freely. The forwards direction guides the head to move forwards on the atlas (C1) as if you are minutely knodding your head affirmatively. It is not forwards in space, like moving the face forwards when peering at the computer screen, but rotating the head forwards by only a few degrees at the AO joint. The upward direction of the head is always so that the crown of your head moves away *from the spine.*

Allow the back to lengthen and widen

When the spine lengthens, it helps it become longer, reducing any over-curvature of the spine that may have occurred through misuse. When people first think about lengthening the spine, a narrowing of the back can often occur. This narrowing is sometimes known as over-arching the lumbar region or pulling the back in. Thinking of the whole back widening simply prevents pulling the back in.

This primary direction is simple and straightforward. However, because of our 'unreliable sensory appreciation', it can be confusing when first practised, which is why hands-on lessons are so important. When results do not happen immediately, people presume that they are doing something wrong or the Technique is not working. It is important to be patient and observant, and realize that changing an ingrained habit takes time. It is strongly advised that when people start giving directions, they have at least a few lessons from a registered Alexander teacher to make sure they are progressing in a way that is likely to result in success.

When performing the constructive rest exercise explored in the last chapter the following directions can be very helpful. These need to be repeated from time to time throughout the exercise:

- Allow your neck to be free.
- Think of your head going forwards and up, away from your spine.
- Allow your back to lengthen and widen onto the ground.

- Think of your shoulders releasing away from one another.
- Allow the right shoulder to move away from the left hip.
- Allow the left shoulder to move away from the right hip.
- Think of your knees pointing up towards the ceiling.

It is important to remember that your patient must not do anything or try to find the right position, as the emphasis for this practice is on doing less. The directions listed above are just a few suggestions you can give your patients, but there are many more. If you decide to have a few Alexander lessons yourself, you will be in a better position to know which patients would benefit from the Technique. One basic idea is to gently allow one part of the body to move away from another part. Alternatively, a person can think of a part of their body quieting or muscles softening. Both will encourage muscular tension to release. It may take a few days or weeks before they feel comfortable with this new way of thinking, so please ask your patient to be patient!

CHAPTER EIGHT SUMMARY

- Alexander used mental thought to cure his voice problem long before anyone had heard of neuroscience.
- Our thoughts are much more powerful than many people realize.
- Directing means projecting particular thoughts that people can give to themselves in order to release harmful tensions.
- It is essential not to *do* the directions as this will result in more tension. Just thought alone can transform health.
- Sometimes directions need to be repeated many times before the body responds to the messages, because our habitual tendencies are very strong.

Release into Movement

*As soon as people come with the idea of unlearning instead of learning,
you have them in the frame of mind you want.*

(F. MATTHIAS ALEXANDER IN FISCHER 2000, P. 35)

The human body is a truly amazing structure which seemingly defies gravity itself. It comprises 206 bones held together by muscles, ligaments and fascia. Most of the bones are rounded in their design, which means our upright form is in a state of constant balance rather than being in a fixed state. If you look at the skeleton you will see that the hinge joints of the limbs consist of one rounded bone balancing on another rounded bone. This makes the human body one of the most unstable structures on the planet, which really helps movement.

ROCK AND ROLL

There are two very clear examples of this. The first is the hip joint, which connects the femoral head to the pelvis. As seen in Figure 31, the head of the femur is similar to a ball and fits perfectly into the concave surface of the pelvis (acetabulum). Another example is the knee joint, the largest joint in the human body. It joins the lower end (distal) of the femur to the upper end (proximal) of the tibia. You can see from Figure 32 that the curved surfaces of these two bones are balancing on one another. So, the structure of many of our joints is similar to a golf ball balancing on a tee.

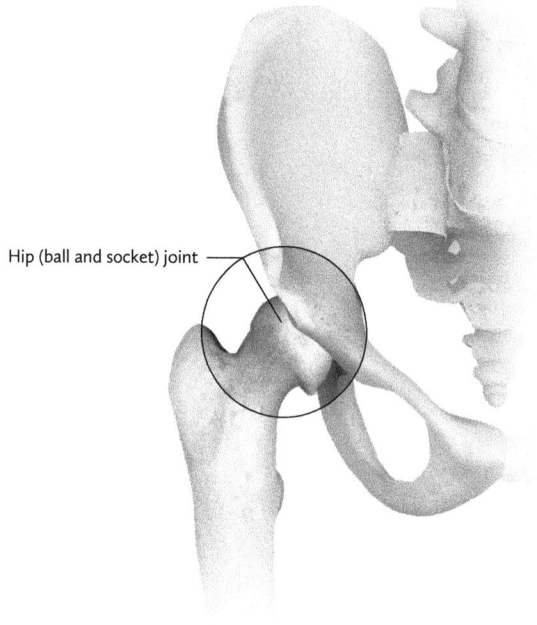

Figure 31: The hip joint is a good example of two large bones joining with one curved surface meeting another curved surface.

Source: Gyer, G., Michael, J. and Calvert-Painter, B. (2016) Spine and Joint Articulation for Manual Therapists. London: Handspring. Figure 2.11A.

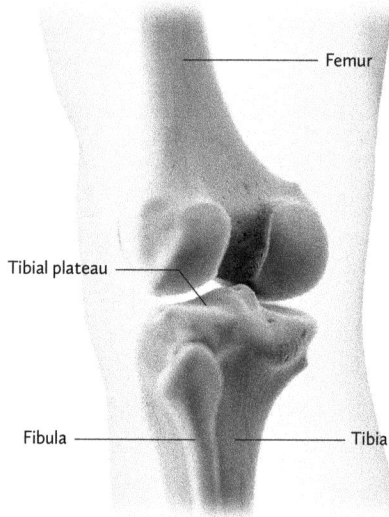

Figure 32: The knee joint is the largest joint in the body, yet it is a 'rocking' joint, allowing the knee to bend easily.

Source: Black, M. (2022) Centred: Organizing the Body through Kinesiology, Movement Theory and Pilates Techniques, 2nd edn. London: Handspring. Figure 2.2.

Now take a look at the other structures and mechanisms that comprise the human form. Let's start at the feet. As seen in Figure 33, the ankle joint also consists of two rounded bones (tibia and talus) balancing on one another.

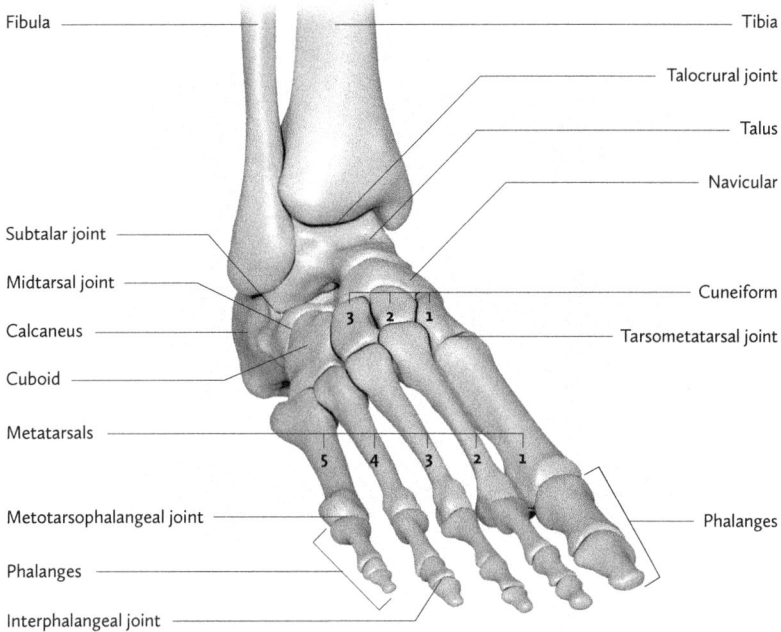

Fibula — Tibia
Talocrural joint
Talus
Navicular
Subtalar joint
Midtarsal joint
Cuneiform
Calcaneus — Tarsometatarsal joint
Cuboid
Metatarsals
Metotarsophalangeal joint — Phalanges
Phalanges
Interphalangeal joint

Figure 33: The ankle joint is a hinge joint with the tibia rocking on the talus.

Source: Gyer, G., Michael, J. and Calvert-Painter, B. (2016) Spine and Joint Articulation for Manual Therapists. London: Handspring. Figure 14.1.

The heel is also rounded, as are the sesamoid bones in the area often referred to as the 'ball' of the foot (see Figure 34).

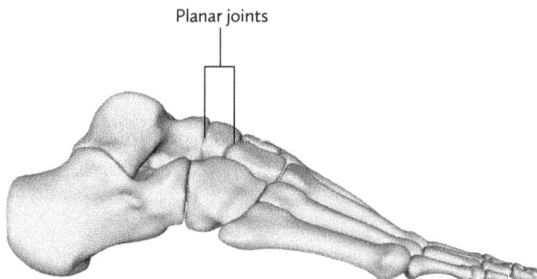

Planar joints

Figure 34: The heel and many other bones of the foot are also rounded in shape.

Source: Gyer, G., Michael, J. and Calvert-Painter, B. (2016) Spine and Joint Articulation for Manual Therapists. London: Handspring. Figure 2.6.

Even the bones we sit on, the ischial tuberosities, are rounded in shape, which allows us to rock backwards and forwards (see Figure 35).

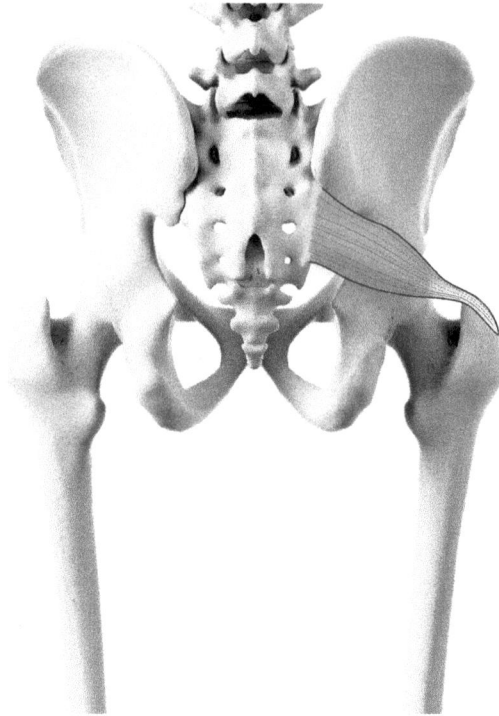

Figure 35: Even the bones we sit on are rounded in shape, which allows easy movement when moving.
Source: Abrahamson, E. and Langston, J. (2019) Muscle Testing. London: Handspring Publishing. p. 162.

The roundedness of many bones clearly demonstrates that we are designed to move easily even when we are sitting. The curved shape of many of the bones does nothing to help stability, but is the first strong indication that we have evolved over many thousands of years to move with little or no effort.

The second indication can be seen in the design of the spine. If you have ever built a tower with children's building blocks by putting one on top of the other, you will know that as soon as you reach the ninth or tenth block the structure becomes very precarious and tends to fall over. In the human spine, five lumbar, 12 thoracic and seven cervical vertebrae (24 in total) all balance one on top of one another. Not only that, but we have evolved with a head which weighs on average between 4.5 and 5.5 kg (10–12 lbs) sitting right on top of that structure; this design makes us top-heavy, which further increases our instability. The AO joint is the place where the skull pivots on the spine and the surfaces of this joint have the same curved shape as seen elsewhere in the human form. The movement of this joint occurs as two rounded occipital condyles of the skull rocking on the superior articular surface of the atlas (C1), which is concave in shape (see Figure 36). As we move, our bones are rocking and rolling on one another, which facilitates easy movement, bringing a new meaning to the term rock and roll!

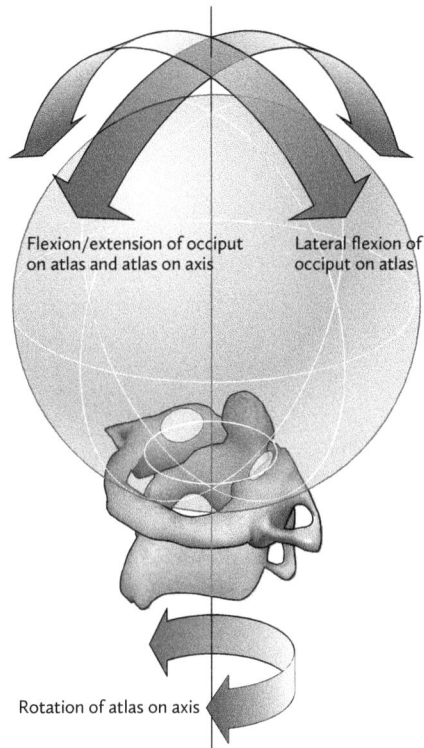

Figure 36: Even our head is designed to rock backwards and forwards on the atlas. The rotation of our head occurs when the atlas (C1) pivots around the axis (C2).

Source: Black, M. (2022) Centred: Organizing the Body through Kinesiology, Movement Theory and Pilates Techniques, 2nd edn. London: Handspring. Figure 9.4.

OFF BALANCE

This brings us to an interesting piece of anatomy that very few people are aware of. The definition of the word *balance* is an even distribution of weight enabling someone or something to remain upright and steady. The pivot point is where an object rotates around, sometimes referred to as the fulcrum or rotational axis. As you can see in Figure 37, the human head is very finely balanced directly above its centre of gravity with powerful neck muscles maintaining that balance. When these muscles release it allows the head to move forwards and up.

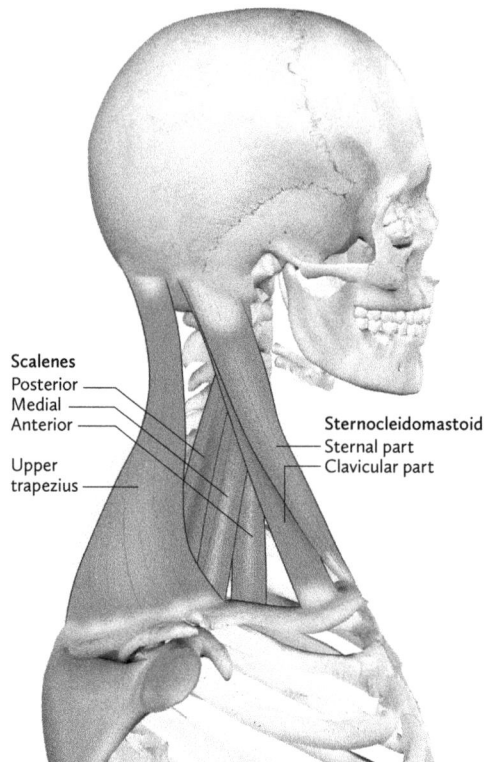

Figure 37: Huge muscles are always supporting our head in all our everyday activities.
Source: Black, M. (2022) Centred: Organizing the Body through Kinesiology, Movement Theory and Pilates Techniques, 2nd edn. London: Handspring. Figure 9.10.

If you watch someone falling asleep while sitting, you will notice that their head often drops forwards and down onto their chest. Just by releasing the tension in the muscles at the back of the neck the head (skull) can move forwards and up effortlessly. If the muscles surrounding the AO joint also release, the head can move freely in any direction. The head then moves *slightly* forwards on the spine in an upward direction, and this slight forwards and up change of the head's position will take the rest of the body into movement as long as other joints and muscles are free.

RELEASE INTO MOVEMENT   101

In other words, in order to move, a human being has only to let go of the tension in certain muscles and our complex reflex systems will do the rest. Many other objects require the most effort to initiate movement. For example, a car or aeroplane needs most power when it accelerates from a stationary position. In contrast, the human body requires no effort to move, in fact, it can move by releasing muscle tension as long as this is not prevented by tension elsewhere. Once the head begins to move forwards, the body will naturally follow, and reflexes are activated as a response to the movement. In short, the way the head balances on the spine in relation to the neck and back controls, organizes and guides all our movements with little or no effort which is exactly how young children move. To me, these are strong indications that we have evolved to move.

SCIENTIFIC RESEARCH

When Alexander prevented the head pulling back, his entire body started to perform differently. He discovered how freedom of the AO joint influenced the movement of the rest on the body, and he named this influence the primary control. The existence of a primary control was scientifically proven in the early 1900s by Rudolf Magnus, a German professor at the University of Utrecht, who was a researcher on the physiology of posture. Magnus discovered a system of reflexes governing posture during a long and detailed series of experiments, which he called 'central control' and which in essence was scientific support of the 'primary control' Alexander had discovered nearly 20 years earlier.

Many people, with the exception of young children, are interfering with their primary control by unconsciously pulling their heads back. This impedes the forwards movement of the body and can interfere with other mechanisms, including respiration, digestion and blood circulation. The primary direction, as described in Chapter Seven, enables the primary control to work without interference. This next awareness exercise can help you observe how the head influences movement.

EXERCISE

- Ask your patient to sit in a chair, then ask them to stand up and sit down again four or five times.
- Watch them carefully from several angles, including the front, the sides and the back.
- If you see their head moving forwards as they rise, notice if they are also pulling it back onto their spine at the same time.
- When you stand behind them, notice if their hair line drops down onto their back. This is a strong indication that their head is retracting back onto their spine.

HOW OUR MUSCLES MOVE US

Muscles can only contract or stop contracting (release) (Figure 38). The contraction of any muscle pulls on the tendon and causes our bones to move, which then act as levers. As one set of muscles contract, the opposite set of muscles lengthen. However, a muscle contraction cannot 'push' the bone back into its original position, and because of this, muscles work in 'antagonistic pairs'. The set of muscles that contracts is called the agonist while the muscle that is relaxing, or lengthening is called the antagonist. Antagonistic pairs swap roles depending on the movement carried out. The agonist is the initiator of the movement, but Alexander realized that it was also possible to relax or lengthen a muscle to initiate a movement. This way of moving takes much less effort than when initiating a movement by contracting, which dramatically reduces wear and tear on the body. I am convinced that this is how we were designed to move.

Doing in your case is so 'overdoing' that you are practically paralysing the parts you want to work.

(F. MATTHIAS ALEXANDER IN FISCHER 2000, P. 39)

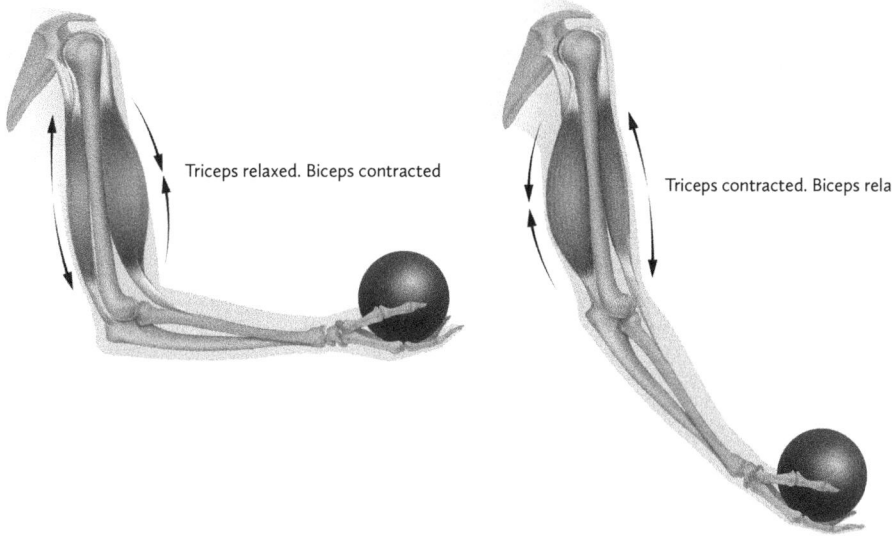

Triceps relaxed. Biceps contracted

Triceps contracted. Biceps rela

Figure 38: Muscles work in pairs so movement can occur as a muscle contracts *or* when a muscle releases.

Effortless movement is evident when watching a young child walking, jumping and running with grace, poise and ease. It is much faster to initiate a movement by tensing, which can be vital when we need to protect ourselves, yet releasing into movement puts the body under less pressure. This next exercise will demonstrate the difference between the two.

EXERCISE

Stand in a room with plenty of space around you and lift an arm out to the side until it is horizontal. Perform the action quite quickly and hold it up for 30 seconds.

1. Notice how it feels and where most of the tension in your arm lies.
2. Put your arm down and let it rest.
3. Raise the same arm quite slowly, thinking of the underside of your arm getting longer.
4. Does your arm feel different the second time? If so, in what way?

So, by people first stopping and thinking before their move they can give themselves a choice of moving with tension or with a release of tension, which can make a big difference to someone in pain. If they tense into movement the condition is often exacerbated, but in my experience, those who learn to release tension to move soon become pain free.

CHAPTER NINE SUMMARY
The human body is clearly designed to move easily because:

- Many of the bones are rounded in shape.
- Joints of the limbs consist of rounded bone articulating on another rounded bone.
- Our structure comprises 206 bones, often one bone balancing on top of another.
- The weight of the head is approximately 5 kg (11 lbs) balancing on top of the spine, making us top heavy.
- We can move easily and freely by releasing muscle tension.

It's All Connected

You translate everything, whether physical, mental or spiritual into muscular tension.

(F. MATTHIAS ALEXANDER IN FISCHER 2000, P. 36)

Everything about us is interconnected. Our muscles do not work in isolation from one another; the muscular system works as a whole. Every system in the body affects every other system and even the way we feel or think affects the way we move. Alexander referred to the inseparability of mind–body as *psycho-physical unity*. He was adamant that mental and physical parts of ourselves are so inextricably united that it is impossible to consider one without the other. Just watch a frightened cat as it tenses all of its muscles simultaneously. Alexander discovered this unification when observing himself in front of the mirror. As he saw his head pulling back, he realized that excessive tension was present throughout his whole body, particularly in his legs and feet. Even his toes were contracted downwards in such a way that it caused his feet to be arched, affecting his whole balance.

If a person goes to a doctor with foot pain, it would be unusual that there would be an examination of the patient's neck muscles to see if the neck was the cause of the problem. Yet, most medical practitioners would agree that a patient's balance can be affected if the head is retracted backwards. Head retraction can cause people to grip the floor with their feet and toes to maintain balance. This is exactly how an Alexander Technique teacher works with their pupils. We do not only look at where the pain or problem is, but rather look at the person as a whole. Learning and applying the

Alexander Technique helps to eradicate the root cause of the problem and so prevents the recurrence of symptoms in the future.

DIAGNOSTIC IMAGING TECHNIQUES

Tools used in evaluating health problems rarely reveal the underlying issue of excessive muscle tension. While diagnostic imaging techniques such as X-rays, MRI, and CAT scans are invaluable instruments for looking inside the human body, they can only identify damage that has already occurred and not what has caused the problem in the first place. I personally find X-ray or MRI reports very useful to see where any problem is located, but then I work out, through touch and observation, the reason for the damage in the first place. Many people come to me with no previous injury or accident; the person reports that the pain they are experiencing seemed to start for no apparent reason and have 'normal' MRIs. However, there is always a reason or cause even if it is not evident. Diagnostic scans can be particularly helpful in cases where habits cause injury, such as a prolapsed or herniated disc, because the direction of the protrusion is a strong indication of the person's habit. For example, if a disc protrudes to the left, it may well mean the patient habitually leans to the right. The primary responsibility of an Alexander teacher is to identify the detrimental habit that is the source of any problem. If, for instance, a patient has a strong habit of leaning backwards when standing, no drug, injection, manipulation, massage, rest or exercise will result in any long-term change.

Pain can often cause a person to tense, and that tension can result in even more pain. Therefore, all forms of pain relief play an important role during a patient's recovery. However, from my own 35 years of experience working with people, merely treating the symptoms without dealing with the root cause usually results in short-term relief, if any at all. If, as a health-care professional or someone involved in the fitness industry, you suspect that that the health issue of one of your patients or clients is caused by harmful habitual movements, yet cannot identify the actual cause of the problem, you may find it useful to refer them to an Alexander teacher for assessment or even work together to help the person. The Alexander work will not interfere with any treatment they are having, because the Alexander work is educational and is not a treatment or therapy.

OTHER SYSTEMS IN THE BODY

As previously explored throughout this book, excessive muscular tension not only affects a person's alignment and biomechanics, but it can affect the actual health and durability of the bones themselves. Sustained pressure on the bones and joints can cause them to wear out prematurely, contributing to osteoarthritis. Osteoarthritis is the most common joint disease in the world. In the summary of the research paper 'Prevalence of diagnosed arthritis – United States 2019–2021' led by Elizabeth A. Fallon (Fallon *et al.* 2023), it states that 20% of adults in the USA suffer with osteoarthritis, while according to the website of Versus Arthritis (n.d.), over ten million people in the UK suffer with the same condition. If a person moves habitually with excessive muscular tension over many years it is likely to result in increased wear and tear of the bones and joints. As a person reduces muscle tension, the pain reduces and movements become freer. Excessive tension can also cause intervertebral discs to bulge or be damaged, as in the case of prolapsed or herniated discs, as was the cause of my own back problem.

Excessive tension in the muscles can also obstruct the flow of blood around the body; when a muscle becomes tense it also becomes harder, which can obstruct the flow of blood, requiring the heart to work harder, placing it under strain. In fact, as we saw in Chapter One, Shaw's angina was also caused by excessive muscle tension; as soon as he learnt how to reduce the tension in his muscles, his angina disappeared and never returned.

Tension in the diaphragm and intercostal muscles greatly interferes with breathing. Many people have little movement in their ribcage because the surrounding muscles are so tense that the mobility of the ribs is restricted, resulting in fast and shallow breathing. In fact, Alexander was known as 'The Breathing Man' because those who had lessons from him claimed that their breathing became slower, deeper and calmer. My pupils often tell me that they sleep better and wake up more relaxed after applying the Technique consistently during the day.

It is a similar story with the digestive system. When muscles are tense, they compress the intestines and stomach, contributing to acid reflux. When muscles are free from excessive tension, a person tends to feel calmer and the action of eating their food becomes calmer and more mindful, which can help a variety of eating disorders.

MENTAL BENEFITS

Mental wellbeing is also helped by learning and using the Technique. As the body and mind are unified, the reduced tension in the muscular system is directly reflected by the mind becoming calmer. By applying the Alexander Technique, many pupils become more confident, enabling them to face the challenges and changes with which they were previously unable to cope. People who are worried, insecure or anxious become less so. In fact, worry and anxiety are mental habits that have been acquired over many years, but by inhibiting and directing, people can let go of these tendencies.

My pupils have reported that their quality of sleep has improved since starting Alexander lessons. Sleep is our natural process for healing and rejuvenation and is a vital component of a balanced and healthy lifestyle. I have known many people whose attitude to life has completely changed so that they now look forward to their day rather than complaining about their lives. People also report that, although the situation at work or at home remains the same, they no longer feel as stressed and consequently have fewer arguments or conflicts. After a series of Alexander lessons, people often mention that their mind is calmer, leading to improved memory and greater efficiency at work. In short, by practising the Technique we are given the ability to enhance our quality of life. If someone can consciously choose to say 'no' to the things in their life that cause them stress, they can improve their own life, and also have a positive impact on the lives of people around them.

EMOTIONAL BENEFITS

In the fast pace of life when it seems that everything has to be done immediately, people's feelings can be buried so deep that they lose touch with the emotional part of their lives. Many of us are living in a dehumanized society where money and social status come before human feelings, and in the sophistication and pressure of the business world people can lose touch with their emotional needs.

By applying the Alexander Technique people become more able to return to a balanced life where emotions and human values once again have the importance they deserve. Through this rebalancing, people replace frustration, anxiety and worry with happiness, peace and harmony. Concern about the future is gradually replaced by an enjoyment of each day as it comes and people will begin to appreciate all the precious gifts they already possess, rather than hankering after material goods, romance or status. When we can absorb and enjoy each and every moment as it comes, then we are truly rich. A person's mind can be thinking of past experiences or planning the future, and their emotions can be experiencing the nostalgia of what has gone or longing for what might be, but a person can never leave the here and now. When your patients or clients can focus on the present moment, they can be truly alive. By using the tools of inhibition and direction, they can experience the miracle each moment brings.

As excessive muscular tension disappears, people often feel that a weight has been lifted off their shoulders. They feel they have more energy and gradually gain more control of their life. They become more able to express their feelings in a constructive way, rather than letting emotions build up and erupt inappropriately at a later date. Past emotions can become trapped within the muscles, and as these release, the emotions are liberated and the person is able to become more balanced. In highly charged discussions or debates, when emotions are running high, the Alexander Technique can be particularly useful.

SPIRITUAL BENEFITS

The Alexander Technique can also heighten a person's awareness, bringing a greater sense of peace to their daily lives. The rush and frantic behaviour are replaced by a greater appreciation of life. They can begin to notice sights, sounds and smells of which they have previously been oblivious. Just consider for a moment what is happening in this very instant – your eyes are reading these words, but you are also breathing. Something is causing you to inhale and exhale, giving you life, and yet this is so often taken for granted. The breath is quietly giving you life each and every moment, but many of us forget to appreciate that quiet miracle that started the moment you were born and continues for every second that you are alive. Behind every breath is your spirit waiting calmly and patiently to be noticed. In short, the Technique teaches a person to be present.

THE BODY HEALS ITSELF

The human body is an amazing healing machine – if we cut ourselves, that cut will heal automatically if the conditions are favourable. This also applies to the harm that undue muscular tension has caused. Once excessive muscular tension is removed, the body will start healing itself. According to Alexander:

> When an investigation comes to be made, it will be found that every single thing we are doing in the Work is exactly what is being done in nature when the conditions are right, the difference being that we are learning to do it consciously.

> (F. Matthias Alexander in Fischer 2000, p. 88)

I want to leave you with a quote from Albert Einstein, which comes from a letter that he sent to Robert S. Marcus in February 1950, explaining the connectedness of all things.

> A human being is a part of the whole called by us universe, a part limited in time and space. He experiences himself, his thoughts and feeling as something separated from the rest, a kind of optical delusion of his consciousness. This delusion is a kind of prison for us, restricting us to our personal desires and to affection for a few persons nearest to us. Our task must be to free ourselves from this prison by widening our circle of compassion to embrace all living creatures and the whole of nature in its beauty.

> (Albert Einstein 1950)

CHAPTER TEN SUMMARY

- The muscular system functions as a whole.
- Excessive muscular tension can interfere with other systems in the body, especially the respiratory, nervous, circulatory and digestive systems.
- Our physical body, mind and emotions are not separate but are inseparable.
- Benefits of the Alexander Technique include:
  - improved sleep
  - calmer mind
  - greater confidence
  - more awareness of oneself and our environment
  - beneficial behavioural change.

The Alexander Technique and the Medical World

Alexander's work is of first-class importance and investigation by the medical profession is imperative.

(DR PETER MACDONALD 1926)

Ever since Alexander made his discoveries, medical professionals and scientists have been divided in their opinion. Those who have experienced the Technique personally were often amazed and astounded by its remarkable effects and would often recommend it highly to their patients. Those without personal experience of the Technique, however, have often dismissed it as unexplainable quackery or perhaps a form of strange hypnotism. When Alexander first started helping people in Australia, several doctors were convinced that Alexander's work was extremely effective, either from their own personal experience or from seeing the effects that the Technique had on their patients. These doctors began referring more and more of their patients to Alexander and he began to gain an excellent reputation for helping with many conditions which were previously considered incurable. A group of doctors, led by Dr J. W. Stewart McKay, a prominent surgeon in Sydney, were so convinced about the international importance of Alexander's discovery that they persuaded Alexander to go to London to present his work to a much wider audience. So, in the spring of 1904 Alexander set sail for London together with letters of recommendation from several distinguished doctors and Alexander prepared himself to give lectures and speeches about his amazing discovery about the primary control.

However, when Alexander arrived in London, he was greeted with a degree of suspicion by many doctors. They could not understand how a man who had never set foot inside a medical school could claim that he could help a wide range of illnesses with one single technique; some doctors thought that Alexander was a charlatan or con man.

Before long, however, Alexander soon gained supporters in the London medical community, especially from R. H. Scanes Spicer, an ear, nose and throat surgeon who took lessons and actively promoted Alexander's method by referring many of his own patients to Alexander. Over time, other doctors became convinced that Alexander had made a discovery that was all-important for good health, including Dr Peter Macdonald, who became chairman of the British Medical Association in 1943. In his inaugural address he declared:

> Alexander is a teacher pure and simple. He does not profess to treat disease at all. If the manifestations of disease disappear in the process of education, well and good; if not, the education of itself will have been worthwhile. Manifestations of disease, however, do disappear. Including myself, I know many of his pupils, some of them, like myself, are medical men. I have investigated some of these cases, and I am talking about what I know. Although the Technique was practically unknown to many doctors, it was of such importance that an immediate investigation by the medical profession was imperative.
>
> *(Peter Macdonald 1989, p. 93)*

Around this time, two other senior surgeons in London hospitals, namely Andrew Rugg-Gunn and James E. R. McDonagh, became lifelong supporters of the Technique and spoke out in favour of Alexander. Rugg-Gunn stated:

> Mr Alexander is an educationist, and not a 'healer' or physical culturist. His teaching embodies with complete precision those principles of psycho-biological behaviour, which are among the most recent

deductions of experimental physiology and applies them in man to a constructive art of living.

(Andrew Rugg-Gunn in McDonagh 1933)

McDonagh, after meeting Alexander and watching him at work, wrote, 'It became apparent to me that the wrong use of the body plays an important role in disease' (McDonagh 1924).

During the 1930s, Sir Charles Sherrington, OM, GBE, PRS, the internationally famous neurophysiologist who received the Nobel Prize in Physiology or Medicine in 1932, became a loyal supporter of Alexander and drew encouraging attention to the Technique by writing in his book *The Endeavour of Jean Fernel*:

> Mr Alexander has done a service to the subject of the study of reflex and voluntary movement by insistently treating each act as involving the whole integrated individual, the whole psycho-physical man. To take a step is an affair, not of this or that limb solely, but of the total neuromuscular activity of the moment, not least of the head and neck.

(Sir Charles Sherrington 1946)

Also, in the 1930s, Professor George E. Coghill, the award-winning anatomist, started to take lessons from Alexander. He too was so impressed with the results that he personally received that he wrote a six-page introduction to Alexander's book *The Universal Constant in Living*. In it he said:

> Alexander seeks to restore the functions of the body through their natural uses. His methods of doing this are original and unique, based as they are on many years of experience and exhaustive study. Yet they can scarcely be adequately described although the results are marvellous... It is my opinion that habitual use of improper reflex mechanism in sitting, standing, and walking introduces conflict in the nervous system, and that this conflict is the cause of fatigue and nervous strain, which bring many ills in their train... Mr Alexander's method lays hold of the individual as a whole, as a self-vitalizing

agent. He reconditions and re-educates the reflex mechanisms and brings their habits into normal relation with the functioning of the organism as a whole. I regard this method as thoroughly scientific and educationally sound.

(Professor George E. Coghill in Alexander 1941, p. xxi)

By 1937, support from doctors had gained momentum and a group of 19 doctors, led by Peter Macdonald, wrote a letter to the editor of the *British Medical Journal* on 29 May declaring:

As the medical men concerned, we have observed the beneficial changes in use and functioning which have been brought about by the employment of Alexander's technique in the patients we have sent to him for help – even in the case of so called 'chronic disease' – whilst those of us that have been his pupils have personally experienced equally beneficial results. We are convinced that an unsatisfactory manner of use, by interfering with general functioning, constitutes a predisposing cause of disorder and disease, and that diagnosis of a patient's troubles must remain incomplete unless the medical man when making his diagnosis takes into consideration the influence of use upon functioning.

Unfortunately, those responsible for the selection of subjects to be studied by medical students have not yet investigated the new field of knowledge and experience which has been opened up through Alexander's work, otherwise we believe that ere [before] now the training necessary for acquiring this knowledge would have been included in the medical curriculum. To this end, we beg to urge that as soon as possible steps should be taken for an investigation of Alexander's work and technique.

(Peter Macdonald et al. reproduced in Alexander 1986, p. 16)

The outbreak of the Second World War in 1939 put a stop to any further investigation. In the 1940s, the first medical research on the effects on the Alexander Technique was conducted by Dr Wilfred Barlow MD, a consultant rheumatologist at Guy's Hospital in London, UK. He was so inspired with Alexander and his technique that he trained for three years to become an Alexander teacher. His research involved photographing a person before and after Alexander lessons standing in front of a grid. The grid helped to measure the dramatic postural changes that took place as a consequence of learning and applying the Technique. Another part of his research involved using an electrical device that recorded activity in neck muscles before and after Alexander re-education. He was able to prove that there was far less activity in the neck muscles after a course of Alexander lessons. A good summary of Dr Barlow's research can be found in his book, *The Alexander Principle* (1990).

It was also around the same time in Boston that Professor Frank Pierce Jones of Brown University approached Alexander's brother for help. Jones had been continually plagued with fatigue and muscular aches and pains and after his initial lesson said:

My first experience of making a habitual movement without habitual effort seems as vivid to me now as it was when A. R. Alexander demonstrated the Technique to me in 1938. Perhaps it was the element of surprise that made the experience so memorable. I had expected something quite different – to have my faults of breathing and voice production diagnosed and to be given a set of exercises to correct them. Instead, Alexander chose the movement from sitting to standing for his demonstration. He made a few slight changes in the way I was sitting (they seemed quite arbitrary to me, and I could not remember afterwards what they were), then asking me to leave my head as it was, he initiated the upward movement without further instructions. Before I had a chance to organize my habitual response, the movement was completed, and I found myself standing in a position that felt strangely comfortable. I was fully conscious throughout the movement, and it was a consciousness of, not of being moved by somebody else – Alexander appeared to be making no effort whatever – but by a set of reflexes whose operation I knew nothing about.

In addition to the reflex effect, the movement was notable for the way time and space were perceived. Though it took less time than usual to complete the movement, the rate at which I moved seemed paradoxically slower and more controlled and the trajectories that my head and trunk followed were unfamiliar. The impression was that of a sudden expansion in both dimensions, so that more time and space were available for the movement. The most striking aspect of the movement, however, was the sensory effect of lightness that it induced. That feeling had not been present at the start, nor had it been suggested to me; it was clearly a direct effect of the movement. While it lasted, everything I did, including breathing, became easier. After a short time the effects faded away, leaving me, however, with the certainty I had glimpsed a new world of experience which has more to offer than the limited set of movement patterns, attitudes and responses to which I was accustomed.

(Frank Pierce Jones 1997, p. 7)

From that first lesson, Jones became fascinated with what had caused that lightness of being, physically, mentally and emotionally, which is one of the hallmarks of the Alexander Technique. Professor Jones dedicated much of the rest of his life to scientifically explaining and verifying the underlying basis for the obvious beneficial effects of learning and applying the Technique, and the research that he did at Tufts University, Massachusetts, USA, which took almost three decades to complete. Professor Jones did many scientific studies attempting to explain how and why the Alexander Technique has the results that it does. During his extensive research, he used multi-image photography, electromyography, force plates and X-ray photography, publishing over 30 papers. During that time, he also corresponded with teachers, scientists and doctors all over the world, and collected a large body of research data. The result was an extensive and fascinating scientific record of how the Alexander Technique works. These studies showed that using the Alexander Technique could produce a marked reduction in the stress on muscles. His results are included in his book *Freedom to Change: The Development and Science of the Alexander Technique and Collected Writings on the Alexander Technique* and are also documented at the Dimon Institute, New York, USA.

Another milestone for the Technique occurred in 1973 when an Oxford professor, Nikolaas Tinbergen, was awarded the Nobel Prize for Medicine and Physiology. He was having Alexander lessons at the time and was so impressed with the results that he devoted half of his Nobel prize acceptance speech to Alexander's work, stating:

> This story of perceptiveness, of intelligence, and of persistence shown by a man without any medical training, is one of the true epics of medical research and practice ... we already notice, with growing amazement, very striking improvements in such diverse things as high blood pressure, breathing, depth of sleep, overall cheerfulness and mental alertness, resilience against outside pressures, and also in such a refined skill as playing a stringed instrument. So from personal experience, we can already confirm some of the seemingly fantastic claims made by Alexander and his followers, namely that many types of under-performance and even ailments, both mental and physical, can be alleviated, sometimes to a surprising extent, by teaching the body musculature to function differently... Although no one would claim that the Alexander treatment is a cure-all in every case, there can be no doubt that it often does have profound and beneficial effects – and, I repeat once more, both in the 'mental' and 'somatic' sphere.
>
> *(Nikolaas Tinbergen 1973)*

ATEAM RESEARCH

At around the turn of the century another event took place in the south of England which was to change the way that doctors viewed the Alexander Technique. The wife of Professor Paul Little developed significant functional back pain in her 30s. Professor Little had heard of the Alexander Technique and encouraged her to have some lessons. Due to the fact that the Technique had made a significant difference to her back pain, Professor Little proposed a major research study to the National Health Service (NHS) to observe the effects of the Alexander Technique. This was a randomized controlled trial (RCT) of Alexander Technique lessons, exercise and massage (ATEAM).

It has been one of the most significant and extensive pieces of research ever carried out in connection with the Alexander Technique and it resulted in the Technique being adopted by the National Institute for Care Excellence (NICE) guidelines which advise doctors on the best evidence-based management of medical conditions. The primary aim of the ATEAM study was to evaluate the effects of Alexander Technique lessons, exercise and massage on chronic and recurrent back pain. The multi-centre clinical trial funded by the Medical Research Council and NHS Research and Development fund was led by general practitioner (GP) researcher Professor Paul Little, University of Southampton, UK, and GP Professor Debbie Sharp of Bristol University, UK, and the results were published in the *British Medical Journal* in 2008, which made news around the world (Little *et al.* 2008).

The trial took nearly a decade to complete as a total of 579 patients with chronic/recurrent non-specific low back pain were recruited from 64 general practices and were randomly allocated to four interventions: six Alexander Technique lessons; 24 Alexander Technique lessons, six sessions of therapeutic massage, or control group. All patients continued to receive usual GP care during the trial. Half the participants also received a GP prescription for general exercise with behavioural counselling from a practice nurse. The Alexander teachers involved used hand contact together with verbal explanation and advice in order to educate the participants' awareness of their postural support and movement patterns. Two main self-reported outcome measures were used: (a) the Roland Morris disability score, the 'industry standard' outcome measure for back function and (b) days in pain in the past four weeks. Ten other outcome measures were also used.

The results of the trial clearly demonstrated that taking individual hands-on lessons in the Alexander Technique led to long-term benefits: following 24 lessons, the number of days in pain was three days per month, compared with 21 days for the control group (an 86% reduction), one year after the trial started, and significant improvements occurred in function and quality of life with a 42% reduction in Roland Morris disability score of those who had 24 lessons compared with the control group. Of the approaches tested, Alexander lessons provided the most benefit, with the 24-lesson group achieving the best results.

Interestingly, the effect of massage on the Roland Morris score was no longer significant after one year, while the effect of Alexander lessons was maintained, the trial authors concluded that the long-term benefits of taking lessons are unlikely to be due to placebo effects of attention and touch and more likely to be due to active learning and application of the Alexander Technique in daily life. Finally, reassuringly, there were no adverse effects whatsoever reported in the trial by any of the 288 participants in the Alexander Technique groups.

Due to this research the Alexander Technique is coming to be better known in the UK and a growing number of doctors are starting to confidently refer some of their patients to Alexander teachers. In fact, in the UK, lessons in the Technique in 2024 may be covered by the NHS in certain locations.

Even more recently, there was a very interesting pilot study (Reddy *et al.* n.d.) where medical surgeons themselves took part in the research; the object of the trial was to examine the impact of the Alexander Technique in improving posture and surgical ergonomics during minimally invasive surgery (MIS). The study was conducted during 2009 and 2010 at the Cincinnati Children's Hospital Medical Center where seven urologists were given an eight-day intensive course of Alexander Technique lessons; these were taught by Jennifer Roig-Francolí and Lois Cone, both Alexander certified by the American Society for the Alexander Technique (AmSAT). The aim of the study was to discover whether training in AT could help improve the surgeons' posture and co-ordination while performing laparoscopic surgical skills.

'The goal of our research is to prove beyond doubt that the Alexander Technique works to improve surgical ergonomics and proficiency so that it can be incorporated as part of graduate surgical training,' said Pramod P. Reddy, MD (Reddy *et al.* n.d.), lead investigator and director of Pediatric Urology at Cincinnati Children's. 'Minimally invasive procedures require surgeons and assistants to maintain awkward, non-neutral and static postures of the trunk and extremities. This limits the natural shifting of their posture and can lead to discomfort, fatigue and even injury (Reddy *et al.* n.d.).

The subjects were tested in many different areas before and after the training. Results of the training programme showed statistically significant improvements in overall posture and specifically upper body and shoulder endurance. Without exception, all the surgeons experienced subjective improvement in their overall posture and a definite reduction in discomfort while performing MIS manoeuvres. The study clearly showed that further study is warranted as it points to the possibility that Alexander Technique training for surgeons could help reduce surgical errors related to surgical fatigue syndrome and also reduces the number of repetitive strain injuries to which MIS surgeons are prone. The research was published in *The Journal of Urology* in 2011 (Reddy *et al.* 2011), was presented at two major US medical conferences in 2010, and won second prize for clinical research papers from the American Academy of Pediatrics in 2010.

In recent times, more and more doctors are publicly praising the Alexander Technique, as you can see from the following examples (SASTAT n.d.):

The Alexander Technique stresses unification in an era of greater and greater medical specialization. Its educational system teaches people how to best use their bodies in ordinary action to avoid or reduce unnecessary stress and pain. In enables clients to get better faster and stay better longer. This is undoubtedly the best way to take care of the back and alleviate back pain.

Dr Jack Stern, spinal neurosurgeon and founding partner
of Brain and Spine Surgeons of New York, NY, USA

The Alexander Technique remains the best of the self-care strategies to prevent the sequel of poor posture and poor breathing.

Harold Wise, MD, PC, New York, NY, USA

Lessons in the Alexander Technique taught me how to sit in a state of lumbrosacral poise, and my chronic low back pain gradually became cured. The Technique is true education. Compared to surgery (e.g. for low back pain or for chronic obstructive lung disease) a course of instruction is inexpensive.

John H. M. Austin, MD, Professor of Radiology; Chief, Division of
Radiology, Columbia-Presbyterian Medical Center, New York, NY, USA

The Alexander Technique makes sense in that appropriate use of the body will lead to reduction of various musculoskeletal disorders and remediate others which are established. No equipment is needed, just the skill and training of the teacher. This technique is very worthwhile as a primary preventative therapy. It is especially useful when posture is a key factor in back injuries while lifting and for workers who perform repetitive tasks while sitting.

Robert D. Greene, MD, Emergency Department,
Norwalk Hospital, Norwalk, CT, USA

I recommend people to the Alexander Technique who have not improved with traditional rehabilitative therapies. Part of their pain may be due to posture and the improper use of their bodies. Many people who have neck or back pain and have gone through heat, ultrasound and massage with no relief can be helped by learning the Alexander Technique. It definitely works. Nothing works for everyone. As one well-versed in using physical therapy and biofeedback, I know how valuable this technique is. I highly recommend it.

Barry M. Schienfeld, MD, Specialist in Rehabilitation Medicine and
Pain Management, Community General Hospital, Harris, NY, USA

The Alexander Technique can help relieve pain and prevent recurrences by correcting poor posture and teaching proper patterns of movement.

Andrew Weil, MD, American physician and author

Testimonials of Those Health-care or Fitness Professionals Who Have Had Personal Experience of the Alexander Technique

A few years ago, Kieran Tobin, a medical consultant, came to see me because of an ongoing neck problem; he was the senior surgeon at the University College Hospital, Galway, Ireland, and had been the president of both the Irish Otolaryngological Society and the ENT section of the Royal Society of Medicine of Ireland. He was also a senior lecturer for the medical students in their training to be doctors. He was kind enough to write a short account of his experience:

> At around the age of 40 years, I began to have problems with neck pain and restricted neck mobility to the extent that it was interfering with my work as an ENT surgeon. As the years went by the problem was sometimes quite bad and I had to manage it with the use of painkillers and other treatments from time to time, but these only gave me short-term relief. An MRI merely showed the expected wear and tear changes.
>
> On retirement I had anticipated relief, but this was not the case. Instead, the pain became quite an intrusion on my life and the limited

mobility meant that I couldn't turn my head, but had to turn from the waist instead.

A friend suggested that I tried the Alexander Technique and, at first, I was somewhat sceptical that anything was going to work, but I can only describe the relief gained, and maintained, as quite incredible. With the help of a local Alexander teacher, Richard Brennan, within a very short time I was back to being quite mobile and virtually free from pain.

Since then, I have attended Alexander Technique sessions on a two-monthly basis for several years and I have been comfortable most the time. Unfortunately, a few years ago I developed an abscess on the intervertebral disc between C6 and C7 which was due to a dental source and required surgery and stabilization. Despite this setback, continuing with Alexander lessons kept me quite well. However, I still had a mild stoop, and although after my Alexander sessions I always felt taller and lighter, the stoop returns after a few weeks. Without my regular sessions, I am convinced that this stoop would have become much more pronounced causing me serious pain whenever I moved my head.

After consulting my Alexander teacher again, we decided that a concentrated period of sessions over several consecutive days would probably be beneficial. I had four daily sessions initially and after a break of five days this was followed by a further three daily sessions. At the end of the time my posture had improved tremendously to the point that the stoop was gone completely. I still have occasional discomfort in my neck, but 90% of the time I am entirely pain-free. I believe doctors and medical students should have far greater awareness of the Technique's many benefits.

(Kieran Tobin, senior surgeon at the University
College Hospital, Galway, Ireland)

Jack Stern, MD, PhD is a board-certified surgeon specializing in neurosurgery and is co-founder of Spine Options, which is New York's first and only facility committed to non-surgical care of back and neck pain. He wrote the following introduction to Deborah Caplan's book entitled *Back Trouble* (1987). Deborah Caplan was a physical therapist in New York City who was also an Alexander teacher.

Back trouble is a frustrating problem for both patient and physician. Physicians are trained to relate signs and symptoms to specific diseases and to diagnose and treat accordingly. But in the case of chronic back pain, it is often impossible to make a specific diagnosis, and most treatments fail. The patient, increasingly dependent on analgesics, gets frustrated and depressed, and the physician loses tolerance for the patient he cannot treat. As a result, more than ninety percent of patients in chronic pain clinics are there because of back pain.

The impact of back pain is felt not only by physician and patient, but by society as a whole. The cost of medical care and of absenteeism from the workplace amounts to many billions each year – yes, billions. Back pain is the most expensive disease of the middle-aged worker.

What is even more alarming is that the number of people who have back trouble is increasing while our understanding of the condition remains inadequate, and our treatment haphazard.

Can the situation be changed? And how?

Let me start by saying that little will change until the medical community becomes open-minded about legitimate alternatives to conventional – but usually unsuccessful – medical therapies. The Alexander Technique is one such alternative. It is a system for teaching people how to best use their bodies in ordinary action to avoid or reduce unnecessary stress or pain. It is a system of postural education, a way of heightening the kinaesthetic sense.

My own exposure to the Alexander Technique came about quite by accident. As the neurosurgical director of a busy spinal service, I am in constant need for qualified physical therapists who are knowledge-able about spinal mechanics and, equally important, are interested in care of patients with either acute or chronic back ailments. Finding such therapists is difficult, and when one opened her office near the Westchester Centre, I was delighted.

What amazed me about this new therapist was that her office con-tained only a chair and a table with a mat, yet the patients I sent her were getting better faster. I soon discovered that she was teaching them how to use their bodies with the ease of movement for which the body was designed and intended. Oh yes, she gave them specific exercises, but most importantly, she used the Alexander Technique.

Well, up until that point the only Alexanders I had been familiar with were Alexander the Great and Alexander's Ragtime Band. F. M. Alex-ander was a new acquaintance. It is not my objective to tell you about him or the Technique since you have bought this exciting book. I will say, however, that the uniqueness of the Alexander approach is that it emphasizes using the mind and body in unity. This is undoubtedly the best way to care for the back and alleviate back pain.

The Alexander Technique stresses unification in an era of greater and greater medical sub-specialization. It enables patients with back trouble to get better faster and stay better longer.

(Jack Stern, MD, PhD in Caplan 1987)

The former GP and medical editor of this book, Dr Miriam Wohl, was inter-viewed by *The Association of Sports & Exercise (BASEM) Journal* (Wohl 2017). This is an extract from that interview.

Dr Wohl: Why is the Alexander Technique in the NICE Guidelines (UK)?

Answer: Because, unlike physiotherapy, osteopathy, chiropractic, Pilates, yoga and supervised exercise, only the Alexander Technique has been shown in a large randomized controlled trial published in a peer reviewed journal, to provide substantial long-term benefits in chronic low back pain. 590 people were studied and had on average 21 days per month in pain. One group had normal GP care (painkillers, physiotherapy, etc.) and at the end of the year they still had 21 days in pain. One group had six sessions of therapeutic massage (which provided the same amount of time and touch); at the end of the year, they had on average 19 days of pain. Another group was advised to take exercises (half an hour of brisk walking or swimming daily) and at the end of the year they had 14 days in pain (this is consistent with other RCTs of supervised exercise in low back pain). Another group was prescribed the exercise after attending six Alexander lessons; at the end of the year, they had ten days in pain. The last group attended a full course of 24 individual Alexander lessons (and half of them were prescribed the exercise). At the end of the year, they had three days in pain and those who did the prescribed exercise gained no advantage. Not only is there RCT evidence for the efficacy of learning and applying the Alexander Technique in chronic low back pain, but the Technique is also in the NICE guidelines for Parkinson disease after an RCT showed statistically significant benefits in the performance of the activities of daily living and in depression scores for people on drug treatment for Parkinson disease.

Question: Evidence for benefits in other conditions – how is this achieved and what is the relevance for sports and exercise?

Dr Wohl: It is because learning and applying the AT enhances general functioning that is so beneficial in back pain, and improves the performance of daily activities in people with Parkinson's disease. Similar enhancements have already been shown in pilot trials for such diverse conditions as performance anxiety and blood pressure lowering in musicians, respiratory function, balance in elderly people, knee osteoarthritis, neck pain, gait, chronic pain, stuttering, postural tone and surgeons' posture.

Question: [Is the Alexander Technique] Alternative or Orthodox?

Dr Wohl: Many so-called 'alternative' or 'complementary' therapies (as well as recently some of the very popular painkillers) have fallen from favour once properly conducted trials or reviews have shown to be a little or no better than placebos (cf paracetamol), but each time the microscope or scientific enquiry has hovered over the Alexander Technique, the results have been positive, all without any gruesome side-effects (cf ibuprofen). As a former GP, nothing I've learned in 33 years of studying the Alexander Technique is at variance with orthodox medicine and science. Further research is ongoing and the published results are promising.

(Dr Miriam Wohl 2017)

Žiga Repanšek was a professional Slovenian basketball player, forced to retire early from a serious sports injury. He was helped back to health by the Technique and now helps others as a sport and somatic trainer using the Alexander Technique. This is his story:

One of the first things I remember in life is running around the block and the soccer ball I got for my fourth birthday. For as long as I can remember, I loved playing and moving. The biggest punishment was that I had to sit still. The legs twitched and kicked, almost of their own accord, wanting to enjoy the movement. I believe that the need to move is innate in all living beings. Movement is absolutely necessary for survival, for the preservation of the species. The desire to move is therefore placed in our cradle and is one of the bases from which other abilities (cognitive, emotional) develop. I mean movement in the widest possible context and not sport, which represents only a small part of movement activities.

As a child, I practised many sports: skiing, swimming, athletics, handball, volleyball and soccer. At first, I trained in two or even three sports at once. I was in love with any game, with movement. At the age of 11, I started practising basketball and later happily devoted almost all of my free time as a teenager to it. The training sessions were first organized two times a week, then three times, and after a good year I trained in basketball five times a week. This is how I came from a spontaneous child's game to 'real training' – special basketball training focused on results.

What followed was years of 'normal sports training', repetition of special basketball elements, exercises for strength, speed, co-ordination and precision. Exercise after exercise, all to reach the desired goal. Children's spontaneous playfulness and the joy of movement gave way more and more to focus on one goal. Win and become the best.

To this day, I can't determine when I started to lose my spontaneous playfulness, but I still enjoyed training in basketball, which is why I enrolled at Faculty for sports after finishing high school. I successfully studied there and was at the same time playing basketball professionally in Slovenia at the highest level in many international competitions.

Due to the way I trained and focusing exclusively on the result, I have been injured many times. Sprained ankles, strained muscles and ligaments, and back pain were a constant. If the injury was not too severe, I still trained most of the time, despite the pain. With a little less intensity, but so much more caution. So, I started using unnecessary and ineffective compensatory movements with muscles that were not created for the optimal way of movement. Over time, I unknowingly changed the way I had moved as a child. Inefficient movement has become my habit. But I didn't know at that time that when a person loses the innate gift of natural and effective childlike movement, it is extremely difficult to get it back later.

In that period, I still firmly believed that there is no success without pain. In a way, I longed for the feeling of exhaustion from training, because I was sure that this was the only way to reach the goal, to success, to victory.

When I look back today, it's no wonder that with such an approach to training and attitude towards myself, I soon seriously injured my knee. Even before the injury, but even more so during rehabilitation after knee surgery, I began to feel severe pain not only in my leg, but also in my lower back.

Due to injuries and pain, I had to end my sports career, and at the same time, I also began to severely limit the amount of movement, as I was constantly afraid of renewed pain in my spine and knee. The pain was sometimes so bad that I couldn't get out of bed or put on my socks in the morning.

My only goal became avoiding more pain no matter what I did. I got caught up in thinking that I had to avoid certain positions and movements so that the tension and pain wouldn't increase. In this way, I completely changed the way I moved, and movement became more and more ineffective and stiff. Occasional pain thus became chronic pain.

When I got caught in the trap of chronic pain, the main problem was no longer just physical pain, which to some extent I got used to, but psychological defence mechanisms began to play an extremely important role too. There was a fear that the pain would return. So, the negative cycle of pain perpetuated itself.

The paradox is that during this time I completed my studies at Faculty of sport and obtained the official title of sports teacher. In other words, I was awarded the highest certification in the country as a movement teacher. It was years later that I asked myself, 'How is it possible that I was able to get an official document for a movement teacher who will teach physical education to children – given the fact that I myself, more than clearly, cannot and do not know how to move effectively?'

For many years I lived and taught physical education with chronically tensed back muscles. I regularly did exercises for back stabilizers and sit-ups and tried to maintain basic fitness because I firmly believed that this would help reduce my pain. I visited many orthopaedists, physiatrists, physiotherapists, personal trainers, kinesiologists, occupational and manual therapists and all kinds of healers; however, I could not get rid of chronic tension in my back. After nearly two decades of stiff movement, knee pain and chronic back pain, my back completely failed during a stressful time in my life. I underwent emergency surgery for a herniated disc in my spine and the resulting paresis of my leg. After the operation, I felt like a porcelain statue, completely stunted, with broken movement co-ordination and a clumsy gait. I was learning how to walk again. I remember for a few weeks after the surgery I was back to working out and training every day, walking up the stairs and doing exercises to maintain my strength and at least minimal fitness. But with such an approach, I only reinforced extremely bad movement patterns and accumulated even more pain and even more tense muscles, which I could not relax even at rest.

It was only a few months later, when the already bad condition practically did not improve and I still could not feel part of my leg and foot, I realized the approaches of sports training and physiotherapy known to me, which are mostly based on increasing strength and exercises to stabilize the trunk, were more than obviously not helpful. Despairing again of my spastically stiff leg and painful back, I began to look for alternatives. First through the practice of mindfulness, my path led me to Hanna Somatics and the Feldenkrais method. Both methods are based on awareness of movement and finding different ways of performing movement. Especially with Feldenkrais, I learned how to explore movement – and movement became play again. I have been researching and combining methods for several years. A few years later, however, I discovered the Alexander Technique, which completely fascinated me. I will never forget the unusual, but wonderful feeling of ease after my first lesson, so every time I travelled abroad, I looked for Alexander Technique teachers there and went to lessons, because there were no teachers in Slovenia at that time. However, the Alexander Technique became more interesting with each lesson or workshop I attended, because I experienced firsthand how successful it is in reducing tension and pain in the body and in changing harmful habits. I was so impressed with the Technique because of its effectiveness that I quit my job in Slovenia and moved to Ireland with my family and enrolled in the Alexander Technique training programme.

By using myself more effectively, I not only managed to reduce the tension in my body and eliminate chronic pain, but I also started to perform many movement tasks again, which I had not been able to do for more than a decade. I hadn't dared to do them. One such is squatting and crouching. When I learned to direct myself better, I realized that my spine will not 'explode' if I do a squat. When I squatted for the first time in more than ten years at the Alexander Technique workshop, I started to cry with joy. Slowly, the fear of pain and other psychological limitations that I built up during and after the injury began to melt away. And when I started to reduce the fear of pain and injury, the tonus in the muscles started to decrease; I allowed the extension of the spine more easily, which enables energy-optimized movement. The cycle of chronic pain, fear and negativism began to turn in a positive direction.

Over time, I have become more attentive to the way I get up from a chair and how I sit down, I am more aware of how I stand, walk, swim, or wash dishes or sweep. Life is no longer a bunch of urgent tasks and activities that I carry out because I once got used to it or because I was told by parents or teachers or heard from the coaches that it's just the right way of doing it.

When I walk to work, go for a walk with the children or go for a run in the forest, I can do it more mindfully – I am more aware of myself and the world around me. I have improved perception by paying attention to how I walk and exploring different ways of walking. I 'play' how I can put my foot on the ground in a different way or how I can direct myself differently.

The next principle of AT, which helped me a lot, is the mental attitude towards the process of the activity I am carrying out. In this way, it is easier for me to focus only on the process of performing the movement and not only on the result. So, I began to realize again that there are many ways in which I can perform a movement in a different way and not direct myself into movement purely out of the automatism of habit. The most important thing is that with a changed mental attitude, I started to enjoy movement again. And when I started to really enjoy movement, movement became a game again.

When I intend to do somatic, Feldenkrais or any other motor exercise, I can now choose how and in what way I will do it. I used to do these exercises automatically – I would lie on the floor with the goal of feeling better and do the exercises. While performing the exercise, I would try hard to quickly explore all possible movements, while impatiently waiting for when I would be able to perform a certain pose or asana perfectly. Or when would I finish the last series of exercises for the trunk stabilizers. My mind was focused only on the goal – the potential result of the exercise – but not on the process of carrying out the exercise – the activity.

Today, I lie down in a similar way, except that I am more aware of the process of performing the exercise and know how to pause several times during the activity. This way, I can direct my movements better, I pay more attention to how I intend to move, and above all, I don't rush as much as I used to. Even before I lie down on the floor, I stop for a moment and think how I could do this according to Alexander Technique principles. So, I no longer lie down on the floor automatically, out of habit. In this way, it is easier for me to choose directions and to decide more easily how I will lie down and also, in what way I want to perform any exercise.

Before public speaking or before talking to students at school, I stop from time to time and think about freeing the neck and allowing the spine to lengthen and widen and only then start to talk. Sometimes I take a short active rest before a speech or performance, other times there is no time for that, so I exhale a few times after the Alexander Technique breathing procedure.

Before I start walking, I stop for a moment and allow freedom in my neck. The nose almost invisibly nods forwards, and at the same time I point my head up which allows the direction of my head to lead the rest of my body into movement – into walking or running. Softening the muscles in the neck makes it easier to direct the head forwards and up, thus gently pulling the spine behind it, and legs reflexively follow the movement of the head and torso. I don't need unnecessary muscle tension for my movement, but let the movement be controlled by reflexes, which allow the most efficient use of energy during a 'controlled falling into walking'. When walking, I don't need to excessively tense the muscles of the legs and lean heavily on the standing leg to lift the other leg to make a step forwards. I also don't need to raise my shoulder unnecessarily when writing, typing, speaking or reaching for a glass on the table.

The Alexander Technique offers me tools to ground myself more easily and find the centre of gravity within myself. Using the basic principles of the Technique allows me to pay attention and slow down more easily when I find myself rushing through life again, when there's no need to. The Alexander Technique showed me that every activity I perform can be an opportunity for a different, more effective response. In this way, I can choose my reactions more freely and have more control over myself. I no longer need to do exercises to improve or maintain my fitness; I no longer have a bad conscience about not doing 'exercises' for my abs and deep back muscles on a daily basis. I don't run any more just because I haven't run for two days or because I think I will be out of shape due to physical inactivity. Today I run when I want to run and at a pace that suits me today. No bad feeling about how fast I think I should run and how many miles I think I should run. Much more important than the end result is the process and the way I perform something – how I direct myself in movement and how I can walk through life more easily. I have experienced that I can choose the way I move, as long as I am not too burdened with the goal I want to achieve or with mental wandering.

By introducing the principles of the Technique into everyday life, I not only help myself, but can also bring knowledge to students at school in physical education classes. I used to teach and evaluate students by rigidly following the knowledge criteria for various sports disciplines. Today, however, I devote most of my time to injury prevention and encourage students to find the movement they enjoy, with the main goal of making them fall in love with their body and movement.

Pain and injuries are a part of life, and most people would like to find an immediate solution to their problems. I myself was no exception. I looked for solutions in doctors and healers of all kinds, but I never thought that the solution to my problems lay within me. The path to this realization was not easy. I perceived the pain, the inability to move easily and the diagnosis as a cruel blow of fate that took away the life I was used to. I felt sorry for myself and often asked myself, 'why me?' Today I can say that injuries, diagnoses and pain have been my best teacher – perhaps the only teacher who was able to change my thinking and was the reason for radical changes in my life. The Alexander Technique opened the door to a new life for me; it taught me conscious control over my movement and behaviour, which allows me to move more easily and have more freedom in my responses to life's challenges.

(Žiga Repanšek)

Elisa Asín Senosiáin is a professor of movement at the Conservatory of Music in Pamplona, Spain, helping music students to move with ease and awareness. She has had individual lessons as well as numerous group classes with me over the last ten years. This is what she had to say about her personal experience of the Technique:

My teaching has greatly benefited from the Alexander Technique. The understanding that certain habitual movements by the musicians I work with can be harmful is very important. For me, the Technique is not about adjusting static posture, but rather about the observation and improvement of movement during performance. Indeed, I try to help my pupils to think in activity so that they can avoid injury and improve their performance. I usually establish thought sequences for my students before and during their activities such as visualizing and thinking about the movements they are going to make as well as being aware of their actions as they are playing. This is something that helps them maintain attention to details, not only in the most technical exercises but also in the most creative, ones and also allows them to stay relaxed, temporarily setting aside the final result that they intend to achieve.

Furthermore, the Alexander Technique helped me understand that, as long as a person continues to repeat exercises mechanically in order to increase muscle strength, stretch muscles or relieve back pain without self-awareness, their habitual ways will become more ingrained. This will most likely result in further problems and consolidate the harmful patterns that they are precisely trying to avoid. In short, I learned that you cannot improve your body disposition efficiently without becoming aware of your own detrimental habits. And second, the Technique is a unique way of practising any discipline of human movement, with emphasis on our integral being, which promotes calmness and poise in action, which is essential in any musical performance.

I would like to share with you a short anecdote that perfectly describes how the Alexander Technique has helped me personally in the practice of dance, body expression, Pilates and other disciplines, as well as in teaching them to my students. Recently I was on the beach resting and trying to put aside the habit of constantly having my cell phone in my hand. Thanks to this I was able to dedicate myself fully to observing my environment and, especially, the people around me. This is something that I have always enjoyed and consider it to be a great source of learning. Not far away from me was an elegant woman who was sitting on a towel with great presence. She was sitting with her legs crossed in the lotus position of yoga.

She caught my attention because she moved with unusual grace and ease. I immediately thought she would be a specialist or teacher of some somatic technique, and I realized that it was her upright posture and presence in her movements that had captured my interest. I continued to watch her with even greater curiosity as she was going to eat a tangerine. I was mesmerized by the graceful way in which she prepared to peel it.

First, with an unhurried, peaceful and elegant movement, she placed it in front of her with her arms outstretched, while remaining seated and upright. As her long fingers began to remove the peel, I began to wonder how she would eat that tangerine; in what way would she bring it to her mouth? I imagined that she would pick up a segment of the fruit and bring her hand gracefully to her mouth. However, I was really surprised at what happened next: she actually took her mouth towards the tangerine, pulling her head back with a lot of force as she pulled her head right back and strained her neck and, in that moment, lost all of her balance, co-ordination and grace.

Then I thought, there we have it, a completely unconscious habit; an everyday habitual movement that most people make completely unconsciously. I wondered then how much time and effort it would have taken her to achieve that striking poise and elegance. Yet, she threw it all away in one second of 'end-gaining'. If you are reading this and know about the Alexander Technique, you are probably able to recognize why the anecdote is so relevant. This is one of the main lessons that the Alexander Technique taught me, the value of observation: first, before performing any action, and second, during the action itself. This is because the awareness at the precise moment can detect any harmful movement, which helps to discover what is needed to prevent the interference with our natural movement. The role of the Alexander teacher is simply to help us recognize these harmful habits which by ourselves we are unable to perceive.

(Elisa Asín Senosiáin)

Professor Joan Van Dyke is a professor of dance at Indiana University of Pennsylvania. She deals with all forms of movement on a daily basis and uses the Alexander Technique principles in her work.

Learning and applying the principles of the Alexander Technique can provide professional and dedicated dance teachers with new and effective approaches to pedagogy for all levels and age groups of dancers.

Training and teaching ballet for over 50 years has allowed me to develop body awareness through movement. The combination of repetition in a ballet class along with a sophisticated understanding of proprioceptive and kinaesthetic awareness provides the perfect environment to integrate the Alexander Technique with ballet training. As a professional dance teacher, training in the Technique in Galway, Ireland, I have been able to identify the process of the integration of the Technique to dance.

When I started the 1600-hour training course, I intended to explore and apply the AT method to my movement awareness in everyday life. I then began to practise integrating some of Alexander's principles into my teaching of dance, particularly ballet. This included inhibition, not to be goal orientated, and being aware of my faulty sensory awareness. While somatic practice is typically associated with modern dance, the highly stylized and competitive dance genre of ballet can be performed with more ease of movement, which frees the dancer to explore more artistic expression in performance when integrating principles of the Alexander Technique.

One of the most difficult and important concepts to teach, especially to young children, is 'alignment', and 'placement' in dance. The Technique allows teachers to address these concepts from a holistic perspective. The principle of allowing the head to move 'forwards and up', which leads to a transfer of weight distribution, is found organically and therefore easier to access.

In dance, we often talk about 'gripping' or 'muscling' our way through a particular movement, which, over time, can affect other body parts and movements, sometimes causing overuse injuries that could have been avoided. Through the understanding and integration of the Alexander Technique, dancers are given additional options of approaching any particular movement; this helps to increase the success and joy of movement in both beginners and advanced levels. The added benefit of injury prevention and awareness lends itself to the quality of movement and longevity of a career or lifestyle of dance.

Another area that I discovered while exploring the integration of Alexander principles in the pedagogy of ballet was the ballet class, which although done in a large group format can feel isolated. While this isolation is necessary for artistic interpretation, there are times during the class that allow room for student interaction through observation, touch and, if there is time afterward, discussion. I have applied some simple AT exercises to the prescribed 'barre work' format involving student interaction. I have noticed an enjoyment within these interactions that could lead to a team/company-building framework, a collegial environment, and an overall positive and more welcoming experience. Ballet often gets a bad reputation for being too elite, stuffy or self-absorbing. While ballet requires the ultimate focus and training at the professional level, Alexander principles still apply. The AT can be introduced early on in the training of young dancers, and many levels and age groups can experience the joy of ballet while creating a welcoming environment.

(*Professor Joan Van Dyke*)

Kecia Chin graduated as an Alexander teacher in New York in 1999. Ten years later she trained as a yoga teacher and uses the combination of both principles in her New York yoga practice.

Alexander claimed that his technique could improve anything you do, and that is so true when it comes to yoga. I find that my yoga students who also have learnt and apply the principles of the Alexander work are far more aware of their bodies and are much less likely to use unnecessary force to achieve the asanas (yoga postures). They also tend to be more present during the class and much more likely to be aware of their breath during each part of the movements. One of the fundamental principles of the Alexander Technique is to prevent any immediate impulse to react and create a space where a person can determine the best way of achieving a goal; to me this is perfect for those doing yoga as it enhances and elevates the quality and presence of both body and mind moment by moment.

I was already a teacher of the Alexander Technique when I started to learn yoga and I noticed I was able to embody the asanas more independently and with less effort than other people in my class who were beyond my level. Most importantly, I was moving as a whole, rather than just moving my body as just different parts as one is often instructed to do. Incorporating the principles of the Alexander Technique I was aware of and appreciated the interconnectedness of the whole body. The Technique also helped me to identify certain postural habits that hinder the practice of yoga and by changing these habits I was able to release into movement rather than increasing muscular tension. In the Western culture we often try too hard at many things we do; this doesn't work in yoga as the main objective is *to promote health and well-being, facilitating personal growth and self-realization.* Last, I have found that using the Alexander Technique during yoga practice greatly helps to prevent injury and increases calmness of body, mind and emotions. I have found the combination of the two is very effective indeed.

(Kecia Chin)

Resources

USEFUL WEBSITES

Richard Brennan has a private practice in Galway and is the director of Ireland's only Alexander teacher training course, also in Galway. He travels extensively in Europe and the USA giving talks and running weekend and week-long courses. For details of these please visit his website: www. alexander.ie.

For details of an Alexander teacher or group class near you please refer to the websites of the international societies of teachers of the Alexander Technique listed below, which give details of how to find a teacher near to you. All teachers listed on these websites have undergone extensive three-year training.

Argentina
Asociacion Argentina de Profesores de Tecnica Alexander (AAPTA)
https://asociaciontecnicaalexander.com.ar

Australia
Australian Society of Teachers of the Alexander Technique Inc. (AUSTAT)
www.austat.org.au

Austria
Gesellschaft F.M. Alexander-Technik Osterriech (G.A.T.OE.)
www.alexander-technik.at

Belgium
Belgian Association of Teachers of the Alexander Technique (AEFMAT)
   www.aefmat.be

Brazil
Associacao Brasileira da Technica Alexande (ABTA)
   http://abtalexander.com.br

Canada
Canadian Society of Teachers of the F. M. Alexander Technique (CANSTAT)
   www.canstat.ca

Denmark
Den Danske Forening af Laerere l F.M Alekxander Teknik (DFLAT)
   https://alexanderteknikidanmark.dk

Finland
Suomen Alexander-tekniikan Opettaja (FINSTAT)
   https://finstat.fi

France
L'Association Francaise des Professeurs de la Technique Alexander (APTA)
   www.techniquealexander.info

Germany
Alexander-Technik-Verband Deutschland (ATVD)
   www.alexander-technik.org

Ireland (both Republic and Northern Ireland)
The Irish Society of Alexander Technique Teachers (ISATT)
   www.isatt.ie

Israel
Israeli Society Teachers of the Alexander Technique (ISTAT)
   www.alexander.org.il

Mexico

Asociacion de Profesores de Alexander Technica de Mexico (APTAM)
   https://aptamexico.com

Netherlands

Nederlandse Vereniging van Leararen in de F.M Alexander Techniek (NEVLAT)
   https://alexandertechniek.nl

New Zealand

Alexander Technique Teachers' Society New Zealand (ATTSNZ)
   www.alexandertechnique.org.nz

Norway

Norwegian Society of Teachers of the Alexander Technique (NFLAT)
   www.alexanderteknikk.no

South Africa

South African Society of Teachers for the Alexander Technique (SASTAT)
   https://alexandertechnique.org.za

Spain

Asociacion de los Profesores de la Tecnica Alexander en Espana (APTAE)
   https://aptae.net

UK

The Society of Teachers of the Alexander Technique (STAT); STAT is the first and longest-established Alexander Technique organization.
   https://alexandertechnique.co.uk

USA

American Society for the Alexander Technique (AmSAT)
   https://alexandertechniqueusa.org

Alexander Technique affiliated societies

www.alexandertechniqueworldwide.org

OTHER USEFUL WEBSITES

Articles and other information
Websites that include interesting articles and information:
www.alexander.ie
www.alexandertechnique.com

Alexander Technique holiday courses
You can learn the Alexander Technique during a holiday course on the Greek island of Skyros or in Southern Spain. To find out dates contact: www.skyros.com or www.almeji.com.

Posture cushions
Details of good-quality wedge cushions that improve posture for car seats and office chairs.
www.alexander.ie/ATshop.html

Self-help CD/MP3
This audio CD is the perfect accompaniment to this book. It lasts for 40 minutes and talks you through a simple procedure that helps you let go of unwanted muscle tension. This will improve your breathing and posture, and in turn can prevent or relieve backache, neck-ache, headaches and stress. Designed to be used over and over again, benefiting you each time it is played.
www.alexander.ie/audio.html

FURTHER READING

Other books by Richard Brennan

- *The Alexander Technique: Natural Poise for Health* (1991) Shaftesbury, Dorset, UK: Element Books.
- *Stress: The Alternative Solution* (1995) London: Foulsham.
- *Mind and Body Stress Relief with the Alexander Technique* (1998) London: HarperCollins.
- *Change Your Posture, Change Your Life* (2012) London: Watkins Publishing.
- *Back in Balance* (2013) London: Watkins Publishing.
- *The Alexander Technique Manual* (2017) London: Eddison Books.
- *How to Breathe* (2017) London: Eddison Books.
- *The Alexander Technique Workbook* (2022) London: HarperCollins.

Books by F. M. Alexander himself

- *Man's Supreme Inheritance* (2002) Steiermark, Austria: Mouritz.
- *Conscious Control in Relation to Human Evolution in Civilization* (1912) London: Methuen & Co Ltd.
- *Conscious Control of the Individual* (2004) Steiermark, Austria: Mouritz.
- *The Use of the Self* (2001) London: Orion.
- *The Universal Constant in Living* (2000) Steiermark, Austria: Mouritz.

Introductory books on the Alexander Technique

- Chance, Jeremy (1998) *The Alexander Technique.* London: Thorsons.
- Gelb, Michael (1981) *Body Learning.* London: Aurum Press.
- Stevens, Chris (1987) *The Alexander Technique.* London: Optima.
- Nicholls, Carolyn (2008) *Body, Breath and Being.* Brighton, UK: D&B Publishing.
- Park, Glen (1989) *The Art of Changing.* London: Ashgrove Press.

More in-depth or specialized books on the Alexander Technique

- Balk, Malcolm and Shields, Andrew (2006) *The Art of Running: Raising your performance with the Alexander Technique*. London: Collins & Brown.
- Barlow, Wilfred (1973) *The Alexander Principle*. London: Victor Gollancz.
- Barlow, Marjorie (2002) *An Examined Life*. Berkeley, CA: Mornum Time Press.
- Carrington, Walter (1994) *Thinking Aloud*. Berkeley, CA: Mornum Time Press.
- Macdonald, Patrick *(1989) The Alexander Technique as I See It*. Brighton, UK: Rahula Books.
- Maisel, Edward (1969) *The Resurrection of the Body*. Boulder, CO: Shambala Publications.
- Jones, Frank Pierce *(1976) Body Awareness in Action/ Freedom to Change.* New York: Shocken Books.
- Shaw, Steven and D'Angour, Armand *(1996) The Art of Swimming*: *A New Direction with the Alexander Technique*. London: Ashgrove Press.
- Westfeldt, Lulie (1964) *F. Matthias Alexander: The Man and His Work*. Long Beach, CA: Centerline Press.

Other related books

- Bacci, Ingrid (2002) *The Art of Effortless Living*. London: Perigee Books.
- Bacci, Ingrid (2005) *The Art of Effortless Pain Relief*. New York: Simon & Schuster.
- Batson, Glenna with Wilson, Margaret (2014) *Body and Mind in Motion: Dance and Neuroscience in Conversation*. Chicago: Intellect Books UK/University of Chicago.
- Doidge, Norman (2007) *The Brain That Changes Itself*. London: Penguin Books.
- Liedloff, Jean (1975) *The Continuum Concept.* London: Penguin Books.
- Stern, Jack (2014) *Ending Back Pain*. New York: Avery Publishers.

References

Adams Musical Instruments (2014) *Alexander Technique*. Lummen, Belgium and Ittervoort, Netherlands: Adams Musical Instruments. www.adams-music.com/en/news/alexander-technique.

Akerblom, B. (1948) *Standing and Sitting Posture*. Stockholm: A. B. Nordiske Bokhandeln.

Alexander, F. M. (1985) *The Use of the Self*. London: Victor Gollancz.

Alexander, F. M. (1941) *The Universal Constant in Living*. Long Beach, CA: Centerline Press.

Alexander, F. M. (2002) *Man's Supreme Inheritance*. Steiermark, Austria: Mouritz.

BackCare (2005) *Your Back in the Future*. Teddington, UK: BackCare. http://alexander.ie/pdfs/School_Furniture_Report_BackCare.pdf.

Barlow, W. (1990) *The Alexander Principle*. London: Victor Gollancz.

British Chiropractic Association (2018) *Back pain experienced more frequently in the UK*. Wolverhampton, UK: British Chiropractic Association. https://chiropractic-uk.co.uk/back-pain-experienced-frequently-uk.

Bronowski, J. (1977) *The Ascent of Man*. Leeds, UK: Book Club Associates.

Caplan, D. (1987) *Back Trouble*. Gainesville, FL: Triad Publishing.

De La Cruz, D. (2017) 'Why kids shouldn't sit still in class.' *New York Times*, 21 March 2017. www.nytimes.com/2017/03/21/well/family/why-kids-shouldnt-sit-still-in-class.html.

Einstein, A. (1950) Letter to Dr Robert Marcus, February 12, 1950. Einstein Archive 60-425. The Library of Consciousness. www.organism.earth/library/document/letter-to-dr-robert-marcus.

Enfield Chiropractic Clinic (2020) *Low Back Pain*. Enfield, UK: Enfield Chiropractic Clinic. https://enfield-chiro.co.uk/low-back-pain.

Fallon, E. A., Boring, M. A., Foster, A. L. Stowe, E. W., *et al.* (2023) 'Prevalence of diagnosed arthritis – United States, 2019–2021.' *MMWR Morbidity and Mortality Weekly Report 72*, 41, 1101–1107. www.ncbi.nlm.nih.gov/pmc/articles/PMC10578950.

Fischer, J. M. O. (ed.) (2000) *Aphorisms*. Steiermark, Austria: Mouritz.

Huxley, A. (1938) *Ends and Means*. London: Chatto & Windus.

Inhibition (2024) In *Useful English Dictionary*. Retrieved 22 October 2024. https://useful_english.en-academic.com/69904/inhibition.

Jones, F. P. (1976) *Body Awareness in Action.* New York: Schocken Books.

Jones, F. P. (1997) *Freedom to Change*. Steiermark, Austria: Mouritz.

Keegan, J. J. (1953) 'Alterations of the lumbar curve.' *Journal of Bone and Joint Surgery 35*, A(3), 589–603.

Little, P., Lewith, G., Webley, F., Evans, M., *et al.* (2008) 'Randomised controlled trial of Alexander Technique lessons, exercise, and massage (ATEAM) for chronic and recurrent back pain.' *British Medical Journal 337*, a884. www.bmj.com/content/337/bmj.a884.

Macdonald, P. (1926) 'Instinct and functioning in health and disease'. *British Medical Journal 2*, 3442, 1221–1223. www.bmj.com/content/2/3442/1221.

Macdonald, P. (1989) *As I See It.* Brighton, UK: Rahula Books.

Mandal, A. C. (1974) *The Seated Man.* Copenhagen: Dafnia Publications.

McDonagh, J. (1924) *The Nature of Disease.* Portsmouth, NH: William Heinemann.

McDonagh, J. (1933) *The Diseases of the Eye*. Portsmouth, NH: William Heinemann.

Mental Health Foundation (2018) *Stress: statistics*. London: Mental Health Foundation. www.mentalhealth.org.uk/explore-mental-health/statistics/stress-statistics.

Motion (2024) In *Britannica*. Retrieved 22 October 2024. www.britannica.com/science/motion-mechanics.

Mouritz (2022) *The right thing does itself*. Retrieved 24 January 2025. https://mouritz.org/companion/article/the-right-thing-does-itself

Reader's Digest (1975) *The Reader's Digest Treasury of Modern Quotations*. New York: Reader's Digest.

Reddy, P. P., Reddy, T. P., Roig-Francoli, J., Cone, L., Noh, P. H. and Gaitonde, K. (n.d.) *The impact of the Alexander Technique in improving posture during minimally invasive surgery*. Cincinnati, OH: Cincinnati Children's Hospital Medical Center. https://alexandertechnique.com/articles/alexandertechniqueposter.pdf.

Reddy, P. P., Reddy, T. P., Roig-Francoli, J., Cone, L., *et al.* (2011) 'The impact of the Alexander Technique on improving posture and surgical ergonomics during minimally invasive surgery: pilot study.' *Journal of Urology 186*, 4S, 1658–1662. www.auajournals.org/doi/abs/10.1016/j.juro.2011.04.013.

Rolf, I. (1989) 'Rolfing: Re-establishing the Natural Alignment and Structural Integration of the Human Body for Vitality and Well-Being.' Published doctoral thesis, Rochester, VT: Healing Arts Press.

Saint Augustine of Hippo (n.d.) *Saint Augustine of Hippo quotes*. https://onejourney.net/saint-augustine-of-hippo-quotes

Schoberth, H. (1962) *Sitzhaltung, Sitzschaden, Sitzmobel*. Heidelberg and Berlin, Germany: Springer Verlag.

Shaw, G. B. (1950) *London Music in 1888–89*. London: Constable.

Sherrington, C. (1946) *The Endeavour of Jean Fernel.* Cambridge, UK: Cambridge University Press.

Siggins, L. (2012) 'Consultant advocates doctors be trained in Alexander Technique.' *Irish Times*, 7 February 2012. www.irishtimes.com/news/health/consultant-advocates-doctors-be-trained-in-alexander-technique-1.458911.

South African Society of Teachers of the Alexander Technique (SASTAT) (n.d.) *Testimonials from doctors, actors and others.* https://alexandertechnique.org.za/what-is-the-alexander-technique/testimonials.

There are unknown unknowns (n.d.) In *Wikipedia.* Retrieved 8 October 2024. https://en.wikipedia.org/wiki/There_are_unknown_unknowns.

Tinbergen, N. (1973) *Nobel Lecture: Ethology and Stress Diseases.* Stockholm: The Nobel Foundation. www.nobelprize.org/uploads/2018/06/tinbergen-lecture.pdf.

Versus Arthritis (n.d.) *The State of Musculoskeletal Health.* Chesterfield, UK: Versus Arthritis. https://versusarthritis.org/about-arthritis/data-and-statistics/the-state-of-musculoskeletal-health.

Wohl, M. (2017) Interviewed in *The Association of Sports & Exercise (BASEM) Journal 40*, 10–11.

Index